Treating Chronic
DEPRESSION

Treating Chronic
DEPRESSION
Psychotherapy and Medication

Daniel W. Badal

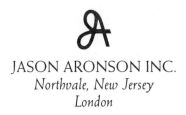

JASON ARONSON INC.
Northvale, New Jersey
London

Information concerning dosages and schedules in this book has been prepared by the author. This information is accurate as of the time of publication and consistent with standards set by the U.S. Food and Drug Administration and the general psychotherapeutic community. As medical research advances, therapeutic standards may change. For this reason and because errors sometimes occur, we recommend that readers follow the advice of a physician who is directly involved in their care.

This book represents the views and opinions of the individual author and does not necessarily represent the policies and opinions of the publisher.

Copyright © 2003 by Jason Aronson Inc.

10 9 8 7 6 5 4 3 2 1

Library of Congress Cataloging-in-Publication Data

Badal, Daniel W.
    Treating chronic depression / by Daniel W. Badal.
      p. cm.
    Includes bibliographical references and index.
    ISBN 0-7657-0330-0
    1. Depression, Mental. 2. Depression, Mental—Treatment. 3. Mental illness—Patients—Rehabilitation. I. Title.

RC537 .B29 2003
616.85'2706—dc21

                    2002071725

Printed in the United States of America. Jason Aronson Inc. offers books and cassettes. For information and catalog write to Jason Aronson Inc., 230 Livingston Street, Northvale, NJ 07647-1726, or visit our website: http://www.aronson.com

Contents

Part I
The Predicament and Its Effect on Chronicity

Part II
Treatment of Chronic
and Refractory Mood Disorders

CONTENTS

List of Figures

ix

List of Tables

Preface

THE PROBLEM:
WHAT THE PATIENT NEEDS

The concepts of chronicity and treatment-resistant depression have become commonplace, and the term "refractory" has entered our vocabulary. Other concepts—quality of life (QOL), subsyndromal, and "spectrum" disorders—have emerged, all of them chronic. The reason is obvious: despite all the new and effective drugs, at least 25 to 35 percent of patients with technically clear-cut mood disorders of one kind or another do not respond in a satisfactory way even though there can be some relief of symptoms. The importance of this is enormous, not only to the individual, but to our culture, as a financial burden to the individual, to the government, to insurers, and also as a major worldwide public health issue (Sartorius 2001). Something has to be done about this. This book is about what can be done with our present equipment. Treatment resistance is to be distinguished from pseudo-resistant patients "resulting from misdiagnosis, unrecognized concurrent medical and psychiatric illnesses, inadequate antidepressant treatment, or unrecognized pharmacokinetic factors interfering with adequate treatment" (O'Reardon and Amsterdam 1998). Pseudo-resistance is one kind of predicament. However, this book will focus on the underlying predicament that causes chronicity in all its forms in patients who are receiving appropriate pharmacotherapy.

This is a small book, but with a large base, namely, the large discoveries in psychiatry of the last several decades, in both biological and psychological psychiatry, and the linkage of the two sciences. By putting the two sciences together in the clinical situation, I hope to describe a way of (1) identifying the problems causing the basic "predicament" of our chronic patients and (2) successfully bringing them back into the mainstream. In the past two decades, many psychiatrists and medical practitioners have relegated the practice of psychotherapy to nonphysician therapists. This is variously known as "split" treatment, or collaborative, combined, or medication back-up (Fawcett 2001).

WHO DOES THE WORK

The medication management of antidepressants has become so complex with these more chronic cases as to require advanced expertise in the field, and a separate book. However, in this kind of "split treatment" the case manager or psychotherapist should have access to enough details and general principles of pharmacotherapy to evaluate the progress and the effects of the medication, and to allow the psychotherapist to communicate intelligently with the person prescribing, if it is someone other than himself, which is often the case. The psychosocial treatment with psychotherapy, management, and advanced rehabilitation techniques has also become complex enough that this volume will emphasize this phase of the treatment and management and will add something more specific to what Haykal and Akiskal (1999) call the "art of management." In this book, the technique of identifying and treating the predicament begins to change the "art" to a science.

The psychopharmacologist, or any professional prescribing the medication, such as a general practitioner, should understand at least enough about the use of psychotherapy in combination with medication to prescribe psychotherapy when indicated. The chief indication with the group of patients under discussion here is chronicity (i.e., the patient may be partially relieved of symptoms but has some chronic problems). In a busy, hurried practice, the physician may not inquire, and the patient may not be given enough time to complain in a short visit. Also, the psychopharmacologist may not be aware of the techniques available to do the kind of psychotherapy needed for these chronic cases. This is one reason why communication is so important between the two persons working with the patient.

Additionally, the psychotherapist may not be aware of the new and complex pharmacological techniques available today as they advance. This area has become so sophisticated that it requires a separate text. So that the psychotherapist will at least be able to identify the medication, I have included lists of the several classes of antidepressants in Appendix I.

Acknowledgments

I would like to thank several persons who not only encouraged me in this work but whose work and research have helped my own concepts in putting this book together. Dr. Pedro Delgado, head of the department of Psychiatry at University Hospitals of Cleveland and of Case Western Reserve Medical School. His meticulous research and work with medication clarifies much in the way of how it can be used with understanding of basic mechanisms. In addition he has shown a great deal of encouragement to the psychotherapeutic approach, including psychotherapists and psychoanalysts in the teaching staff of his department.

The psychoanalytic group of Case Western Reserve Medical School has been very encouraging, providing an atmosphere of acceptance of my ideas, by giving me the opportunity to teach candidates and therapists. I especially want to thank Dr. Norman A. (Drew) Clemens who, in his leadership in the American Psychiatric Association as Secretary, backs psychotherapy and psychoanalysis. In his writing and publishing, he has brought professional attention to basic principles similar to those in this book.

The Hanna Perkins Center for Child Development of Cleveland, famous throughout the world for its work with children, deserves my thanks for the contribution made by the underlying principles of that work to my own concepts underlying the treatment of adults. Thomas F. Barrett Ph.D. the director, and Chair of the John L. Hadden, Jr. Center for Psychoanalytic Child Development has articulated these concepts in a very helpful way.

Special thanks to Dr. Robert Furman and the late Mrs. Erna Furman (Poppy) for their contributions. Their work in the treatment of children and on the development of children is known throughout the world through direct teaching and publishing (eight books on such subjects as "self-control and mastery in early childhood"). They provide valuable insights as to how children's problems can lead to adult problems and even illness. This has been a very important source of corroboration and understanding of the observations I write about in this book.

Finally, I want to thank my family for their encouragement and enduring patience with me as I became very preoccupied in writing this book. . . . They agree that it is worth the time spent to get my message across.

Introduction

A brief encounter I recently had at the local super-market dramatically tells the central theme of this book. Milling around at the vegetable counter, I met a woman I had known for years, the daughter of a couple who were once neighbors and friends. I had seen her 6 or 7 years ago in consultation, at which time she gave a history of anxiety and depressions that had been troublesome and recurrent since her college days but not vigorously or appropriately treated. Because of closeness to the family, I thought I should refer her and sent her to "the best," a very competent psychiatrist who specialized in mood disorders.

At the present encounter, she looked painfully anxious and depressed and immediately gave a quick but troubled account of the current situation, which she summarized by saying, "Everyone is so busy." The original psychiatrist had given her medication, but she seemed not to be helped by a number of well-known antidepressants. They seemed to make her more anxious, and she never had a satisfactory, effective medication. She was now in the hands of a very experienced colleague of the original psychiatrist, and had also just started to see a woman therapist, who, she said did not seem to understand how painfully depressed she can be. In this chance encounter, she seemed to be appealing to me, to be anxiously asking for help. I saw how troubled she was and immediately felt involved and responsible. I responded thoughtfully by suggesting that she should give the new therapist a chance and see what happened in a few visits and that she should definitely let me know how it was going.

But I was troubled by the experience. If in 5 or 6 years of treatment by "the best," she was still so seriously depressed and anxious, then no wonder that the statistics for satisfactory recovery in general were so unfavorable. I had thought that in a paper I wrote over 20 years ago I had described how, with a careful approach, any knowledgeable psychiatrist could in time get over 90 percent of depressed people reasonably well. After the encounter with this woman, I thought, "Is this what is known as a refractory case?" Or is something left out? She was obviously getting the best modern pharmacotherapy and yet was still not well. This was not a pseudo-resistant patient who was being neglected, but an actual refractory depression that needed something more. What more should be added in even the best of current treatment programs for these long-term cases? I feel justified to say in answer," That is what this book is all about." Herein I describe some interesting techniques to add to the current accepted programs that will, I think, increase our success rate with chronic and so-called refractory depressions.

In my own paper on chronicity (Badal 1979a), I reported that after 2 years of intensive treatment, 35.4 percent of treated patients in my closely followed group of 65 were still disabled by depressive symptoms. I discovered and reported that a combination of factors added up to a painful "predicament" that the patient could not solve. This predicament consisted of a combination of two conditions: (1) a very unsatisfactory and painful interpersonal relationship and (2) a serious personality defect, which handicapped the patient's ability to deal with the relationship, creating the predicament. By identifying and treating the patient and his predicament, I had been able, in time, to bring about a satisfactory result in over 90 percent of the patients in the group, leaving less than 10 percent not doing well, most of whom had some serious physical illness, such as cancer under treatment, which dominated the picture. The theme of this book is the definition, identification, and treatment of this basic predicament, which contributes to the cause of the depression and its chronicity.

Since the paper cited above was written, additional evidence has accumulated in my practice, and also in the field, that my conclusions were valid, that such a predicament does exist, but that some cases were complicated by influences in addition to or other than the two I identified in the predicament at that time. Using the DSM-IV Multiaxial System as a basis, I have added to the two original factors as summarized in the following paragraph and given in detail in Chapter 5.

The predicament results from a combination of easily identifiable negative factors such as stress, heredity, comorbidity, personality—a total of 17 factors—balanced against positive factors such as healthy interpersonal relationships, no comorbidity, and lack of character pathology—a total of five positive factors. Using these factors, I have formulated the essentials of a method, using the Multiaxial System to develop a scoring system. The result is a numerical score that identifies the group to which the patient belongs: (1) not refractory, (2) possibly refractory, and (3) definitely refractory. Details of the method are described in Chapter 5, and application of the method in treatment, with examples from practice, is discussed in Chapters 6 and 7.

Since my original observations were made, there has been a great increase, not only in my practice but also in the field in general, in the recognition of factors in the patient's life that could contribute to what I called "the predicament" (after Mazer 1976). These factors can delay the response to medication and contribute to chronicity. As a result, a dramatic change has taken place in the understanding and treatment of mood disorders in the last half decade.

In the last half decade, a number of new concepts have entered the field. First, the concept of *chronicity* has sprung up, based on very convincing follow-up studies, especially that of the Pittsburgh group (Kupfer 1997). These studies demonstrated that continuing treatment beyond the acute phases of an attack of depression prevented recurrences in a high percentage of cases. "What gets you well keeps you well!" Treatment is now not just acute, but must be understood to be in three phases: (1) acute, (2) continuation, and (3) maintenance.

Second, another dimension is now being brought forward that goes beyond the standard clinical symptomatology, called *functioning* or, as Weissman (1999) wrote, "social functioning, drive, motivation, performance, and quality of interpersonal relationships." She pointed out that a significant percentage of people were still not functioning normally even after medication had relieved the general symptoms of depression.

Third, much attention has been given recently to discoveries of the neurophysiologists, such as Nemeroff (1998), who have demonstrated that *early environmental stresses and physiological pressures* can cause lasting neurological network changes. In applying this understanding to the mood disorders, research has revealed that children who have had serious traumas, such as serious losses, are prone to have mood disorders later in life. Thus, treatment of the mood disorder can take into account these long-standing tendencies through the use of psychotherapy.

Fourth, the work on treatment now is emphasizing what are called *"refractory"* and *"treatment-resistant"* cases—cases that do not respond readily to the initial treatment and become chronic by definition.

Fifth, partial syndromes, all of them chronic, are receiving attention—*"subsyndromal"* cases and *"spectrum disorders."*

As a result of the recognition of these concepts, it is now understood that five areas of treatment must be addressed with these cases, as follows:

1. The doctor-patient relationship. In long-term relationships, it is an especially powerful therapeutic factor. This is no accidental function, as I will describe in the histories illustrating recovery. It is a combination of a transference relationship and a reality device with a therapeutic impact. *Psychiatric News* (June 16, 2000, p. 1) noted that "outgoing American Psychiatric Association (APA) President Allan Tasman, M.D., urges fellow psychiatrists to recommit themselves to the primacy of the doctor-patient relationship in psychiatric care."

2. Advanced pharmacological treatment. New antidepressants and mood levelers are available, and sophisticated psychopharmacologists have studied dosage, chemistry, and augmentation with combinations and other medications such as thyroid hormone.

3. Psychosocial interventions of all kinds. Studies have shown the effectiveness of these interventions.

4. Psychotherapeutic programs of all appropriate kinds. Cognitive and interpersonal therapies have been tested most. Numerous studies have shown the effectiveness of even the limited types of psychotherapy, especially when combined with medications. Psychodynamic and psychoanalytic therapy is appropriate for treating long-term problems, especially interpersonal and characterologic issues. Although this is not universally acknowledged, my work demonstrates its effectiveness as reported here. Selection of the appropriate type of psychotherapy requires that it be tailored to the individual needs. Whatever is the basis of the patient's predicament guides the selection of the particular psychotherapy.

5. Rehabilitation programs for chronic patients who have long been unable to function well.

In this book, I formulate an approach to solving the problem of recognition and treatment of all these various types of chronic and refractory mood disorders. I present a method applicable to the chronic and otherwise hard-to-treat mood disorders. The purpose of the book is first to focus on the factors involved in the chronic and refractory cases, the latest techniques in the treatment of the chronic and especially hard-to-treat mood disorders, i.e., depressive illnesses of all kinds, including bipolar—those that are resistant to treatment (refractory), those that become chronic, and those that leave something to be desired in the way of functioning even when there is improvement in symptoms. These cases will be described in terms of diagnosis, reasons for the resistance (i.e., the predicament), and methods of treatment. What all these chronic cases have in common is this phenomenon I have named a "predicament."

This book will not explore the advanced psychopharmacology in great detail, except in individual case examples, but will take up the other issues that prevent the patient from responding sufficiently to the medication, that is, the psychosocial and psychotherapeutic issues. For details of techniques of pharmacotherapy, see the case reports and annotated bibliography. This area has become so sophisticated that it requires a special text. The central purpose of this book is to define, diagnose, and treat the predicament, which occurs in persons whose response to appropriate medication is not totally satisfactory.

Part I of the book deals with the definition of chronic mood disorders and recognition of the predicament. I start with a chapter on the evolution of the concept of the patient's predicament from observations made in my own practice and then go on with Chapters 2 and 3 defining chronicity, refractory, and treatment resistance and identifying these patients. Chapter 4 describes the new concepts and their relation to chronicity. Chapter 5 is the crux of the book, with a special emphasis on a new and practical method of identifying the patients who need the special attention that chronicity demands, using the Multiaxial System of the Diagnostic and Statistical Manuals (DSM-IV-TR™ 2000) to identify the patient's predicament in a new and simple way.

In Part II, I deal with treatment of these chronic patients. Chapter 6 turns to treatment in a detailed way, emphasizing the individual's needs and tailoring the treatment to the individual using the new concepts described in Chapter 4 to focus on those particular needs. The final chapter presents the application and techniques of combined therapy through clinical examples. The clinical examples demonstrate the complicated treatment of the factors leading to the predicament and illustrate the length of time required in the more refractory cases.

The references constitute a separate section at the end of the book. First, I included an alphabetical listing of the references cited in the text. Then, I appended a list of additional references for each chapter, for the use of anyone who wants to delve more deeply into the background and substance of the text.

Often, nowadays, the medication is given by a physician and the psychotherapy by a nonmedical therapist. This arrangement is known as "split" or collaborative treatment and requires extra communication between the two professionals involved.

I

THE PREDICAMENT AND ITS EFFECT ON CHRONICITY

1

The Predicament—
Evolution of the Concept

The title of this chapter requires explanation. "Predicament" could mean either an *effect* of the illness or a *cause*. Actually, I use the term "predicament" as a cause of the chronicity of refractory depressions. The predicament, as I originally defined it (Badal 1979a), arises from a combination of two things, namely, a very serious and troublesome interpersonal situation in the love life of the patient, coupled with a personality problem that renders him or her unable to resolve the situation. This predicament is the central theme of the book. Identifying and treating it usually results in significant improvement or recovery of a previously refractory case. It is my hope that readers will find the concept very useful when treating the troublesome chronic and refractory cases of depression.

It must be clearly understood that the treatment of the predicament is *in addition to* the standard treatment with medication and psychotherapy or counseling and not *instead of* the standard treatment. Therapists and psychiatrists merely need to add this concept to their treatment approach to achieve an increase in cures. The concept falls into the domain of combined treatment. Also, it should be understood that the patient might not be fully aware of the predicament or its significance. It sometimes has to be elucidated by a careful search in the course of history taking and/or psychotherapy. The use of the DSM-IV Multiaxial System (American Psychiatric Association 2000) is helpful in identifying the predicament, if thoroughly and carefully done, as will be described in detail in Chapter 5.

The justification for identifying and treating the predicament is that with the average present standard treatment of mood disorders, good as it is, 30 to 40 percent of persons do not respond satisfactorily (see Chapters 2 and 3). A cause or causes must be sought. Even in the hands of the currently most skillful psychopharmacologists, the percentages of satisfactory response with the new drugs are no better than they were in the era of tricyclic antidepressants of the 1960s to the 1980s. Some improvement in the average recovery rate has occurred since the addition of limited amounts of psychotherapy to accepted programs of treatment, but the percentages are still far from acceptable. Something is left out. I hope to supply at least a part of what is missing with the concept of predicament and its treatment.

Over 20 years ago, I wrote a report entitled "Eclectic Treatment of Difficult Depressions" (Badal 1979b). The term "difficult" in the title of that report actually referred to the depressions that either became chronic, i.e., did not clear up during the initial treatment period and still had some symptoms in 2 years or were refractory or treatment resistant to the usual standard methods of medication and management, in or out of the hospital. At that time, it already had become evident to me upon close scrutiny, i.e., intensive treatment and repeated interviews, that in many cases the patient was in some kind of chronic external environmental stress of personal significance with which he could not cope. As I noted in 1978, this situation might not differ greatly from that in which many people find themselves in life but in *combination* with the patient's personality difficulties it resulted in a predicament that was ongoing, chronic, and persistent, which the patient could not solve.

That report was written at a time when it was first accepted by the psychiatric profession to say:

It is now reasonably well demonstrated that all patients do not recover from depressive illness easily with biological treatment, i.e., medication and/or electroconvulsive treatment (ECT). Some are disabled for long periods, and some chronically disabled. It is also becoming

5

more evident that psychosocial and personal factors must be taken into account as causative factors in depression, and in treatment. Even in severe bipolar illness such factors require meticulous scrutiny, as described recently in a very significant report from the National Institute of Mental Health. [Badal 1979b]

For the 1979 study (Badal 1979a), a group of 65 unselected patients was studied intensively and treated over a period of 4 years. They supplied the kind of personal information about intimate relationships not obtainable in large studies or by the use of rating scales. Of these 65 unselected patients, 23 (35.4 percent) had been (or still were) chronically disabled, i.e., unable to function productively at the end of 2 years. In a significant number, there existed a chronic problem, involving meaningful love relationships in combination with a personality disorder, making for a situation that the patient could not solve himself, a situation that I labeled a "predicament" (Figure 1).

With therapy based on intensive work on the predicament, approximately half of the 23 still disabled after 2 years (N = 11) were no longer disabled, and of the 12 still disabled, 6 had good prognosis for ultimate recovery, leaving 6 (9.2 percent) of the total potentially permanently disabled, mainly elderly (1 patient), those with serious physical disabilities (2), and/or those with serious untreated chronic character disorders (3). The total recovery rate thus was 90.8

Figure 1. The predicament in chronic mood disorders—occurrence of stressors in chronically disabled and not chronically disabled patients.

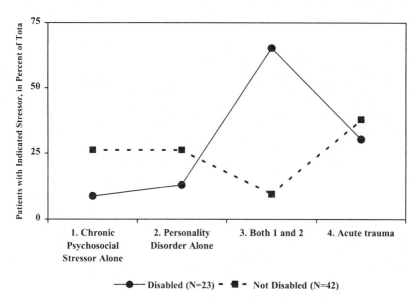

percent in a group of depressed patients, many who had been hospitalized. The key to improvement of the recovery rate was treating the predicament of the refractory cases. Table 1-1 gives the treatments used for this group of patients.

The combination of a chronic reality situation involving love relations and a personality disorder occurred in 15 of the 23 chronically disabled, as against 4 of the 23 never chronically disabled (figure 1) (chi square = 8.97, degrees of freedom (d.f.) = 1, p<0.01). Thus the occurrence of what I have defined as a predicament in the chronically disabled is a significant factor differentiating this group from the group

Table 1-1. Psychological treatments in long-term patients (from Badal 1979a).

Methods	Number of Times Used (N = 23)*
Support, protection	23
Individual psychotherapy; electic therapy	19
Cognitive, educational therapy	18
Interpersonal therapy	12
Insight; psychoanalytic or other intrapersonal therapy	7
Group therapy in hospital	7
Couples therapy (9 married)	6
Spouse treated individually	3
Family therapy	3
Group therapy, posthospital	2
Occupational therapy, posthospital	1
Nursing home	1
Day care hospital	1
Classical analysis	1

*Eleven eventually recovered with integrated therapy of multimodal type

of patients who never became chronically disabled. Of the group of 19 never chronically disabled, 13 had a combination of an unsatisfactory and frustrating reality situation and a personality disorder. However, unlike those who became chronic and malfunctioning, most of these patients had other resources that allowed escape and coping. Those not disabled were able to function and recover with the use of character traits that rescued them.

THE SIGNIFICANT OTHER— ATTACHMENT AND LOSS

My conclusion from this work was that there is a powerful influence in the one relationship in these patients who seem so dependent on one person, in an adult, usually a spouse. However, it can be a parent, a grown child, an employer, etc. When the one person on whom these patients were dependent or to whom there is a deep attachment is not reliable or really available, or worse, lost or absent, the patient becomes depressed to a remarkably disabling extent, much more than just sad. Observations on individuals as well as statistics bear this out. These observations have given rise to the concept of the "significant other," i.e., the person to whom one is deeply attached.

The theory of Bowlby (1969 and 1988) may explain this phenomenon. In his book *Attachment and Loss*, he expressed the theory that in the human animal, as in other animals, there is a need for comfort and support that is essential for development, as are other biological needs such as hunger and sex. The adult's pattern of need is formed in childhood through

9

the nature of the relationship with the parents. Our patients with depressions seem to show that the pattern of their need is transferred to the important significant-other person, whether a spouse or some other, so that a loss of comfort and support is very threatening and depressing. Now, if the person has a genetic biological tendency to depression, he will become depressed when that comfort and support are withheld, whereas another person ordinarily will win back that comfort and support if it is possible, or endure the loss without actually having a depression. Everyone who is unhappy about life does not have a major depression. Our observations on the experiences of our depressed patients often show some recent experience in which actual or threatened loss has occurred.

Understanding the significance of attachment across the life span is also essential to understanding the effect of loss and the pain it causes. A broad description of attachment and attachment theory can be found in a recent general review by Cassidy and Shaver (1999). Loss of an attachment can be particularly important in its relationship to depression as a cause of both acute grief and grief that is prolonged as a failure to complete the mourning process (Zisook et al. 2001 and Badal 2000). Zisook et al. (2001) include many references to the literature concerning both biological and psychological aspects of grief and mourning in relationship to depression.

The healthy mourning process for the loss of the significant other is usually comprised of three phases:

(1) shock, disbelief, or an inability to verbalize the feelings; (2) a process of working through the loss; and (3) replacement with another person or another great devotion. A depression may result if the process is incomplete. For the purpose of this book, the point is that such a loss may be the significant underlying cause of the predicament, and the therapist will have to help the sufferer work through the loss and find someone or something to substitute in order to bring about relief from the depression.

CASE EXAMPLES

(1) Chronically disabled, Example 1

A typical predicament was of a passive person, either man or woman but usually a woman, because of the high percentage of women in the study, married to a man with some kind of problem such as impotence, uncontrollable anger, insensitivity to her needs, or unawareness of her need for some kind of support that he would possibly be able to give if he had insight or motivation. The importance of this situation to the patient also was most significant, but the personality problem was such that he or she could not correct or improve the relationship.

(2) Chronically disabled, Example 2

A man in late middle age with a major depressive disorder of a rather unremitting nature that disabled him totally and required hospitalization for months at a time—a typical agitated, anxious depression of a type formerly called involutional melancholia. Some partial remissions had been induced by electroconvulsant therapy (ECT) and by intensive hospital treatment. His predicament was that he was married to a very ambitious, aggressive, successful businesswoman who constantly put him down, and whom he could not live without because of his great dependence on her. She had completely rejected sexual relations for several years, resulting in his being dissatisfied and discontent; yet he could not either complain or win his wife back, as he felt she was ready to break up the marriage, and he did not dare to take the chance of losing her totally. The situation was thus at an impasse for him, and he was in a submissive position, whereas she was in the dominant one. Her needs were being met better than his, as she could do what she wanted, i.e., to pursue her career and be left alone by him, while his great needs for love and affection and for bolstering his self-esteem were not being met at all. This is a predicament.

Treatment of this kind of person means a great deal of work, not only requiring intensive up-to-date use of antidepressants, augmenting if necessary, plus intensive individual psychotherapy or psychoanalysis plus couples therapy or joint therapy. The fortunate and reassuring outcome is that a sizable proportion of those so treated recover from their chronic disability and invalid state and are able to function again. Therapists of various different backgrounds may have different types of practice and a different selection of patients. Patients in my practice were often referred from someone in practice because they were having too much trouble with too sick a patient. Many of those patients had been sick enough to be hospitalized. To anyone with a psychotherapy practice alone, there would certainly not be as many sicker patients such as this group contained. Nevertheless, this group will represent a population with which most psychiatrists will have to deal.

In Chapter 3, a review is given of the frequency of chronic depressions over periods of 10 and 25 years in order to see whether the occurrence rate in the current study was consistent with and typical of the illness itself. We go on in later chapters to test the current patient population to see whether the concept of a predicament can be found in these patients as well.

2

Definitions and Clinical Description of Chronic, Refractory, and Treatment-Resistant Mood Disorders

DEFINITIONS

This book deals with the chronic cases of mood disorders, focusing on the refractory cases. Almost any mood disorder can be classified in these categories. A good workable definition of chronic depression, based on current categories of DSM-IV, is that given by Rush and Thase (1997): "Chronic depressions include major depressive disorder, recurrent with full interepisode recovery: major depression, dysthymic disorder, and those depressive disorders not specified (NOS) that are persistent or otherwise predictably recurrent with substantial disability." It is important to distinguish among and define the terms "chronic," "treatment resistant," and "refractory." The terms are loosely used in the literature, but in this book the following definitions are used.

Chronic can refer to any long-term illness. For example, most bipolar (formerly manic-depressive) patients have a chronic illness, i.e., one that tends to go on for several years or more, even for a lifetime, although the individual episodes of mania and/or depression can run from a few weeks to a year or two even when under treatment. Bipolar spectrum disorder: In recent years a condition resembling a low-grade bipolar disorder often occurs between definitive bipolar attacks. It has come to be known as bipolar spectrum disorder, and is probably more common than clinically diagnosable bipolar disorders (Hirschfeld 2001). Major depressive disorder is of three chronic types: (1) a single attack of major depression, which can go on for several months to years. The late-life depressions formerly called involutional melancholia lasted a year or two but are terminated earlier nowadays; (2) depression that can recover only partially with acute treatment, or (3) depression that can recover fully but recur. (4) Dysthymia, formerly known as depressive neurosis, tends to be chronic and is sometimes the basis of attacks of chronic major depression.

Treatment resistant usually refers to a single attack of depression or mania that does not respond readily to standard treatment and requires

16

special attention and manipulation of medication, or augmentation by various devices. This is a special field of therapeutics requiring considerable skill and expertise with medication and augmentation. A definition of treatment resistant was recently made by Judd (1999): ". . . there are three major goals in the treatment of major depressive episodes: (1) removal of depressive symptoms (2) reduction or elimination of the associated impairment, and (3) the prevention of episodic relapses or recurrences. Failure to achieve any or all of these treatment goals should be used to define treatment resistant."

Pseudo-Resistant refers to patients who are not getting full and appropriate modern treatment, as described in the preface. Treatment-resistant patients are to be distinguished from pseudo-resistant patients for whom the non-response is "resulting from misdiagnosis, unrecognized concurrent medical and psychiatric illnesses, inadequate treatment" (O'Reardon and Amsterdam 1998). An example is a patient with a schizoaffective disorder of the bipolar type, now in her 60s, who has been in a very well-run but old-fashioned sanatorium for over 15 years because of repeated attacks of psychosis and hypomanic behavior due to noncompliance (i.e., neglecting her medication of lithium and antipsychotics) "because I don't need them. I felt well." During these years she has not had a psychiatrist, but her care is being supervised by a very busy local small-town physician who cannot possibly keep up with the newest developments in the treatment of bipolar illness. She has been receiving haloperidol by needle but has not had an appropriate trial with any of the new atypical antipsychotic medications. As a consequence, she has had symptoms typical of cycling bipolar illness, described by the staff as "talking and complaining all the time, making incredible numbers of phone calls, over-interested in sexual talk, won't go to bed unless we sedate her heavily, etc., etc." I have written the family asking them to get a psychiatric consultation, and a change in medication to the more modern ones now available. She is intellectually well preserved and under ordinary circumstances, now that new mood levelers are available, could probably get considerable more control over the psychosis. This is pseudo-resistant, due to failure to treat properly.

Refractory refers to those mood disorders that have not responded symptomatically to the best of initial treatment with drugs and standard attention (i.e., treatment-resistant cases that even after the special attention of modified pharmacology, augmentation techniques, and immediate attention to environment are still symptomatic). An entire issue of the *Journal of Depression and Anxiety* was devoted to the Treatment of Refractory Depression (TRD) (vol. 5, no. 1, 1997). The definition employed in the lead article, by Berman et al. (1997), is as follows: Treatment refractory is a failure to demonstrate adequate response to an adequate treatment trial, i.e., sufficient intensity of treatment for sufficient duration after all potential factors are then addressed— treatment adequacy, compliance, differential diagnosis, and treatable comorbid conditions. A patient who does not demonstrate a remission may be considered treatment resistant (relative or absolute).

The purpose of this book is to focus on the factors involved in these chronic and refractory cases. The book is not directed specifically at treatment with medication, which would require separate and detailed attention to the drugs. Instead, this book starts where the experts in medication for treatment-resistant depression stop or leave off. The latest techniques in the treatment of especially hard-to-treat mood disorders—i.e., those that leave something to be desired in the way of functioning even when there is improvement in symptoms—will be described in terms of diagnosis, reasons for the resistance, and methods of treatment.

The importance of this group of patients was described recently by O'Reardon and Amsterdam (1998), who note that patients with treatment-resistant and refractory depressions include 10 to 15 percent of those who remain chronically depressed with a significant morbidity and mortality rate by suicide. Fawcett (1994) states that 50 to 70 percent of patients have only a partial response to treatment. Others have said that as many as 50 percent of the patients with a single episode develop a chronic or relapsing course. In one study of 209 women and 161 men followed for 4 years, 43 percent had significant depressive symptoms based on the Global Depressive Scale (Swindle et al. 1998). Predictors of chronic course were: less education, more severe initial depressive mood and ideation, secondary major depression, prior treatment, comorbid medical conditions, and fewer close relationships. Acute stressful life events, marital status, and age did not predict the chronic course, whereas serious medical conditions, particularly cardiac illness, did.

CLINICAL DESCRIPTION
OF CHRONIC PATIENTS

It is to identify and treat these chronic, refractory, still troubled patients—those with some symptomatic relief but with disability or serious problems in functioning—that this book is directed. What do these cases look like clinically? Whom are we treating and for what?

20

In clinical practice, the patients symptomatically fall into several somewhat overlapping but recognizable groups: (1) Those who do not respond satisfactorily or readily to initial treatment within a reasonable expected time, (2) those who respond but have recurrences, (3) those who respond symptomatically as far as the immediate symptoms are concerned, but will be found not to function well, possibly because of personal problems or habits or psychosocial issues, including those with subthreshold symptoms (the so-called spectrum disorders), and (4) those who seem to be functioning in their daily lives but are not themselves satisfied with their recovery, such as their way of performing. The lack of satisfaction can possibly be due to personality issues not apparent earlier. They may have been masked by the illness or lifestyle, and can be helped with more in-depth or specific therapy. Those with phobias or residual obsessive-compulsive symptoms belong here. Some of these patients benefit by psychodynamic or psychoanalytic treatment. There is also a group of patients found to have had the conditions for years, and who were not treated for it; or were treated inadequately, perhaps by a family physician with inadequate medication or with counseling when medication was also needed.

DIAGNOSTIC CATEGORIES

Sometimes rating scales (Sajatovic and Mullen 1999) are very helpful in identifying how sick the patient is at any given time when the depression is not so obvious. They can help in following the course of the illness and in checking progress, sometimes revealing depression when superficially the patient seems well. The two scales used a great deal currently in research are (1) The Hamilton Rating Scale for Depression (Hamilton 1960) and (2) The Montgomery-Asberg Rating Scale for Depression (Montgomery and Asberg 1979).

I have found the self-administered Zung (1965) scale useful at any time before or during treatment for checking the progress of the therapy especially as to how the patient sees himself, an especially important consideration for the depressed or manic person.

In practice, an official diagnosis is necessary for treatment, according to the manual currently in use by American psychiatrists, the Diagnostic and Statistical Manual IV of the American Psychiatric Association (DSM-IV-TR™ 2000), in any one of the following:

Refractory disorders include three clinical groups: (1) official mood disorders, (2) depressive personality disorder, and (3) so-called "spectrum" disorders, meaning partial, not the full disorder. Any of these disorders can become chronic or refractory. Official code numbers have been assigned to disorders included in DSM-IV-TR™ and in the *International Classification of Diseases*, 9th Revision, Clinical Modification (ICD-9-CM). These two manuals give us a working classification based on the clinical picture. The code numbers can be used in reports, thus preserving some degree of confidentiality.

Any of the mood disorders can be chronic or refractory to treatment. Complications such as comorbidity with another illness can make these disorders difficult to treat. The disorder may be symptomatically relieved but the patient can turn out to have disabilities or malfunctions requiring professional attention. We are going to discuss the spectrum-disorder group, as they may be a group in the early stages and therefore vulnerable to chronicity. The main emphasis in this book will be on those with full-blown, definite diagnostic types of categories who have not responded to initial treatment as completely as we could wish. These are either refractory to initial treatment and may have been or will turn out to be chronic or recurrent (respond but recur). The bipolar spectrum disorders are particularly hard to differentiate or to recognize.

HISTORY OF
MODERN DIAGNOSTIC CATEGORIES

The current diagnostic system was arrived at after a great deal of work over several decades. Earlier editions, starting with DSM-I, published in 1952, had been found very useful. It was the first official manual of mental disorders to contain a glossary of descriptions of the diagnostic categories. However, the use of the term "reaction," based on Adolph Meyer's concept of reaction types, as well as the concept of "neurosis" as described by Freud and psychoanalysis, are etiological and developmental concepts and not strictly descriptive, and were given up as official diagnoses. The next editions, DSM-II, DSM-III, and DSM-III-R, were all based on descriptive diagnostic terms that did not imply a particular theoretical framework and are compatible with the *International Classification of Diseases*, 9th Edition, Clinical Modification (ICD-9-CM) (Commission on Professional and Hospital Activities 2001).

These diagnostic categories have been enormously helpful in research and in communication about conditions being seen, and in helping to make judgments about treatment. They do not eliminate etiological research; in fact, these categories allow for more specificity. As stated earlier, the therapeutic process may require uncovering an underlying, unnamed basic factor behind the symptoms as diagnosed here.

HISTORY OF
THE CONCEPT OF CHRONICITY

A generation ago experienced psychiatrists, using the latest in medications and what was considered good and adequate treatment, made remarkably similar observations. The tricyclic antidepressants (imipramine, etc.) worked very well, actually statistically as well as our newer drugs for the most part. Nevertheless, we found then, as we find now, that many patients did not recover fully from their depressions. They might be left with attenuated depression, depressions warded off by drugs or alcohol, regressions in behavior, etc. I published a paper on my observations of these phenomena entitled "Transitional and Pre-psychotic Symptoms in Depression" (Badal 1968). Using psychodynamic concepts, I called these states latent depressions and chronic depressions, with the typical psychology of the depressed patient but with a breakdown avoided by defenses. Latent meant that the depression was still there but covered up by denial, or defended against in some way. I described two main groups:

(1) Characterologic and pseudo-neurotic symptoms—irascibility, chronic obsessive-compulsive personality, projection, and living in fantasy, plus hypochondriacal fixations. This is a stage of successful defense, i.e., successful in that a balance is maintained, although pathological. Latent and chronic depressions belong here and in the next category. [Badal 1968, p. 11]

(2) Regressive phenomena—the use of drugs and alcohol for temporary relief at painful periods—the use of sadistic and masochistic behavior. These are less successful defensive measures, because of ensuing guilt and the complicated problems of addiction. Anorexia Nervosa may fit in here also. [Badal 1968, p. 11]

I also observed what I called prebreakdown phenomena, i.e,

(3) the return of the repressed, uninvited by therapy.

These include frightening impulses, dreams of morbid content, sensory illusions, feelings of depersonalization, and childhood memories (Badal 1968, p. 11).

My summary of these observations was:

There are transitional, non-psychotic and pre-psychotic states of depression, occurring both spontaneously and during therapy. Which way the process goes depends on a variety of factors—environmental influences; the nature of the inner process (as yet not fully explained by present methods); and the treatment employed, i.e., transference influences, chemical (drug) influences, insight. [Badal 1968, p. 23]

Thus the awareness of chronicity has been with us for some time, and psychiatrists working with patients with depressive (mood) disorders over a long enough period of time are not surprised by the current emphasis on the phenomenon in connection with the symptomatic categories of our current diagnostic descriptive categories. But what is the relationship of the descriptive categories (based on symptoms) we use in our work today, to the psychodynamic concept?

Table 2-1 is an attempt to describe this relationship. At the time of my paper (Badal 1968), we were working from a standpoint of development and course as a reaction rather than as a static symptom complex, as it is technically known officially now. In following patients with depression in and out of attacks over a period of time, often years under treatment, it was possible to see the depressions as having a course with variations in symptomatology (i.e., as states belonging to one illness with a full-blown disorder at one point in the course). We also saw that some patients were alcoholic or had other associated problems such as medical illness and could not get well until that problem was solved. Table 2-1 shows the psychodynamics of our current descriptive categories.

Therefore, the recent interest in chronicity does not come as a surprise to those psychiatrists who have been in practice a number of years and have the opportunity to see what happens in the long run to depressed patients. In the paper quoted above (Badal 1968), I reported on several things that demonstrated a kind of chronic linkage among the attacks of depressions any individual has.

Using that concept, for one thing, there were the "watered-down" or partial symptoms of depression that often occur between outright full-blown attacks. Also there are prebreakdown phenomena that showed the return of the repressed, such as being flooded by dreams of the past. There are "regressive" symptoms such as alcoholism and other attempts to control an underlying depression. I also gave a description of the

Table 2–1. Symptomatic and psychodynamic relationships in chronicity.

Current Descriptive Diagnosis DSM-IV-TR™	Psychodynamics
Subsyndromal states	Mourning reaction for past
Spectrum disorders	Defenses against latent depression
Comorbid states, e.g., anxiety	Defenses and regression phenomena
Obsessive-compulsive states	Defensive processes
Prodromal symptoms (memories, etc.)	The "return of the repressed"

unsolicited return of childhood memories, coming like "flashbacks" and reported that this phenomenon can be a prodromal sign of an oncoming serious depression. In intensive therapy, the childhood memories come gradually and are usually preceded by discussion of the childhood history. When they signify an oncoming major depression, possibly a psychotic one, they can come out of the blue, are very vivid, and feel forced on the patient. Anyone in charge of a patient with any of the types of chronicity, either recurrent depressions, or the partial symptoms so characteristic of the long-term intervals, should be on the watch for these phenomena and take steps to help ward off any oncoming downturn, with whatever is appropriate from the therapeutic arsenal such as medication or other treatment moves.

Having become more and more aware of the complex nature of these phenomena that make up chronicity, I decided to look at my practice in the past several decades and obtain some basic statistics on the frequency of chronicity, as it is now defined. The next chapter contains data from my own practice on the frequency of chronic cases, derived from a 25- and a 10-year follow-up, in order to get some actual numbers of what we are dealing with.

3

Chronicity in Practice

How often do mood disorders become chronic? What percentage of the patients in a psychiatric practice is likely to become chronic or refractory? Which types of patients will become chronic? What is the best course of treatment for these chronic patients? To answer these questions, I have reviewed my own practice and experience in this chapter; and in Chapter 4, I have reviewed the current literature for comparison.

The setting of my own practice offers all the current treatment facilities that might be needed in the treatment of any of the broad varieties of mood disorders that are referred to a specialist in psychiatry in a large, modern teaching hospital: access to inpatient service with intensive individual and group treatment, occupational therapy, medical consultation and

treatment by specialists, physical therapy, electroconvulsant therapy if needed, etc. The individual treatment available includes psychotherapy on an intensive
basis as needed, including 5-times-weekly hourly sessions of a standard psychoanalysis if needed. Outpatient services include individual and/or group therapy,
occupational therapy, self-help group follow-up, day
treatment up to 5 half-days a week, and rehabilitation
referrals. The whole process is monitored and directed
by a practicing psychiatrist who forms a therapeutic
alliance with the patient.

The practice also includes referrals by patients
and by psychotherapists, giving the practice a representation of milder and first-time patients. The whole
spectrum of mood disorders is represented in the
practice, and it is not too heavily weighted in the
direction of chronicity. However, it represents a practice on the medical side, with a greater representation
of the standard mood disorders than the practice of a
nonmedical counselor.

To get information from my own patients, I reviewed the records of my practice from May 1975 and
May 1990, and compared them to my patient records
of May 2000. I then calculated the following values for
each of the two periods (10 years, 1990 to 2000 and 25
years, 1975 to 2000):

1. The total number of patients seen and listed.

2. The total number of patients with mood disorders.

3. The number of patients recovered.

4. The number of patients still in contact.

    a. The number of patients in active treatment.

    b. The number of patients not in active treatment but followed and monitored.

5. The number of patients who were deceased.

6. The number of patients whose status was unknown in May 2000.

OBSERVATIONS FROM
THE 25-YEAR FOLLOW-UP

In my practice in the month of May 1975, 17 cases of mood disorder (Table 3-1) were found, of whom 7 were still in active contact in May 2000. Six of those in contact were still on medication. Six additional patients known to have been chronic were deceased, one from suicide. Four cases in psychoanalysis in 1975 are functioning normally out of treatment, although they are known to have been chronic.

Thus, 15 of these 17 patients (88.2 percent) with mood disorders are known to be or have been chronic. Two patients (11.8 percent) have recovered. Four of the patients were bipolar, 1 severe bipolar I. Ten were diagnosed with major depression, and 3 with dysthymia.

Table 3–1.   Summary in May 2000 of 25-year and 10-year follow-up of patients seen in May 1990 and May 1975.

[Of the 17 patients in the 25-year follow-up, about half (47 percent) were still in active treatment. Only 2 (12 percent) were considered recovered and out of treatment. Of the 33 patients in the 10-year follow-up, more than one third (39 percent) are still in active treatment and 7 (21 percent) are recovered and out of treatment.]

	1975 23-Year Follow-Up		1990 10-Year Follow-Up	
	Number	Percent	Number	Percent
Total Mood Disorders	17	100	33	100
Recovered and out of treatment	2	11.8	7	21.2
Still in treatment and doing well	8	47.1	13	39.3
Medication and active psychotherapy	6	35.3	7	21.2
Medication check and 2–4 yearly checks	2	11.8	6	18.2
Deceased	6	35.3	13	39.3
Medical illness	5	29.4	12	36.4
Suicide	1	<0.1	0	0
Out of touch	1	<0.1	0	0

An additional 24 cases were seen in May 1975 but were not followed. Fifty percent of these were mood disorders, making 29 cases of mood disorders in all, with 14 (37 percent) actually known to be chronic cases, of which 8 (20 percent of the total) were still in contact in May 2000 and on medication.

This sample demonstrates that a substantial percentage of the mood disorders in private practice will be chronic. Numbers are important, but the reason for the numbers, the identification of the chronic patients, and what treatments were used are also important. The three examples given below will illustrate typical cases of those who have done well and those who have not done well. The first two examples illustrate the group of patients that are doing well:

The first example is a 70-year-old married professional woman with bipolar II, in psychoanalysis 5 years in her 30s, and maintained on lithium and Prozac (fluoxetine). Very successful in her profession, she amassed a small fortune. She is out of active, intensive treatment but medication is maintained. When she retired at age 65, she had a severe heart attack, recovered slowly, and afterward came back into treatment with weekly sessions. She has gradually resumed a normal life, except that now she is no longer the dominant member of the couple but is dependent on her husband's control of their lives, and she accepts the changes realistically.

The second example is a successful lawyer in his 60s, diagnosed as bipolar II, with very mild hypomanic spells and troublesome depressions once a year. He responds well to increases in medication, originally imipramine but in the last 7 years Zoloft (sertraline). He never has had to stop working but finds that his depressions simply slow him down and temporarily take away his enjoyment of life. He is seen every 6 weeks, winter and summer. Whatever problems he has, mainly interpersonal relationships, are discussed and handled well, without much psychodynamic content. This is an example of the bipolar II cases that are chronic but under good control and simply need medication management and ongoing, mainly interpersonal, psychotherapy 6 to 8 times a year.

The third case is a not-so-happy example of a patient who was allowed to go her way and not checked as regularly or as frequently as she now would be. She was very competent in her professional life and seemed to be doing well personally. This is a woman now (2000) in her 60s, divorced, never remarried, who raised three children by herself. She has a successful professional career and still works. She had two recurrent severe depressions in her 30s for which she was hospitalized. For 25 years, she had been maintained on modest doses of tricyclics with occasional psychotherapeutic visits when she had a personal problem. A major depression spell occurred recently following a severe attack of pneumonia for which she was hospitalized. She had stopped her medication after several years with no depressions. Thus her depression was much more serious than usual and required several months of intensive therapy to bring her back to her normal functioning.

It is quite apparent that patients with recurrent depressions, even those with long periods of normality, should be seen regularly, every month or two. The patient described above should have had more regular follow-up and supervision, but there is something more important with this patient, namely, her personality. She had a tendency to project and to fight with anyone who did not agree with her. She had to have her way. She was not on speaking terms with her siblings, for example, and blamed them for it. Her personality problems were not considered problematic at the outset of her treatment. In retrospect, it would have been helpful if she had had intensive psychodynamic therapy, or preferably psychoanalysis, and had been able to develop more intrapsychic controls over her interpersonal relationships.

This patient illustrates the concept of a core problem—a predicament—behind the symptomatic picture, no matter what the descriptive diagnosis. To understand the patient's personal problems, one has to have some idea of what the predicament is. With this patient, it is a long-standing personality characteristic that has given her much strength in her career but has caused conflicts in her personal life severe enough to cause pain and depression. In the beginning, we did not take this problem into account because she was functioning so well in other areas, e.g., work. The concept has the potential of simplifying long-term care because it allows one to focus on the important issues in therapy. The method of diagnosis I describe in Chapter 5 will simplify the process and enable the predicament to be diagnosed early.

OBSERVATIONS FROM
THE 10-YEAR FOLLOW-UP

For purposes of identifying factors leading to chronicity and its treatment, I also reviewed cases seen 10 years before May 2000. The following numbers represent a 10-year follow-up of the patient roster from May 1990 (Table 3-1).

Of 33 patients with mood disorders in treatment in May 1990 who have been followed, 13 (39.3 percent) are still being actively treated with medication, 13 (39.3 percent) are deceased (12 from medical reasons and 1 from suicide), and 7 (21.2 percent) are out of treatment and doing well. All 33 are known to have been or are still chronic.

Of the total of 49 patients seen in May 1990, including those out of touch, a substantial number are still in treatment and doing well, i.e., 13 (26.5 percent of the total both in and out of touch). Another group is known to be doing well and are in touch, although not in active treatment (9, or 18.4 percent). This makes a total of 22 (44.9 percent) that are doing well. Thirteen (28.6 percent of the total) are known to be deceased and another 15 patients (30.6 percent) are out of touch.

In the 10-year follow-up study, it is difficult to be sure of the actual proportion of the original group that

38

became chronic because the 30 percent of the group who are out of touch could be partly chronic patients or could be recovered. However, the 26.5 percent of the original group known to be chronic, in treatment, and doing well, represents a substantial proportion of the original group. We can say that in the 10-year follow-up, at least a quarter of the original group became chronic and probably more, including some of those out of touch.

It appears that my clinical experience carries out the statistical studies and that one quarter of the total patients seen will require at least 10 years of prolonged treatment to do well. Some will need to be in treatment indefinitely. Another 18 percent have finished their treatment and are doing well.

Two examples will illustrate patients who after 10 years are functioning well. The first example is a patient who is still in active treatment after 10 years and doing well. She is a middle- to late-middle-aged schoolteacher, a widow, who was forced to retire from her job because of heart disease aggravated by the stress of dealing with the physical aspect of classroom teaching. She continues to use antidepressants regularly in moderate doses but has an active social life and is an active grandmother. She is seen monthly to maintain this status.

The second example is a patient who is doing well and is not in active treatment. He is a retired banker in his 60s who is very active in the community in volunteer work. He was hospitalized for a depression in his 30s and then was in active treatment for 6 years, with medication and classical psychoanalysis of 5 days a week. Following the analysis he remained on medication for 10 years, with no recurrences of depression, and for 15 years has been out of treatment altogether and doing well without medication.

PSYCHOANALYSIS AND INTENSIVE PSYCHODYNAMIC THERAPY

Of the 6 patients in analysis 25 years before this writing (1975), 5 have done very well (one of the five has died of heart disease). One patient stopped analysis after 1 year and went to a mental facility on the East coast. My impression is that psychoanalysis has a very good chance of bringing about a great improvement in all cooperative patients, even in some of those with bipolar disorder, both I and II. Typically, these patients still will need medication, even when personality problems have been relieved by analytic work.

Of the 13 patients still in active treatment after 10 years, the 4 who have had intensive (once a week) psychodynamic psychotherapy or psychoanalysis plus counseling are doing very well and are functioning well. Seven of the others have had a good therapeutic relationship, have been in continuous contact, and are functioning well, although they need supportive contact regularly (once monthly) and are on medication. That leaves 2 patients who are on medication and not functioning satisfactorily personally although able to work. One of these is doing well except in personal relations.

The impression is that the psychoanalytic therapy and its derivatives such as psychodynamic therapy are very helpful in bringing about an improvement in the interpersonal and social functioning. Also, the person of the psychiatrist-therapist appears to fill a need these formerly depressed persons have, and does not just administer drugs. This person may represent an auxiliary "self" for the patient, and appears to be helpful in the prolonged cases, once chronic or refractory, and now functioning very well. Of the 12 deceased patients, 11 died of unrelated medical illness and 1 of suicide (a bipolar II who committed suicide when both his wife and his psychiatrist were out of town). This case illustrates the importance of the "significant other" in the lives of the chronic patients.

SUMMARY OF FOLLOW-UP STUDIES

These follow-up studies of the 25-year and 10-year groups of patients would seem to indicate that the group of patients diagnosed with mood disorders in the last 1 to 3 decades has contained substantial numbers of patients whose illness was chronic despite the discovery and use of the latest pharmacodynamic method and drugs.

The inescapable conclusion from my observations and corroborating work (Badal 1979a and b) is that if we are to help the chronically disabled, we must identify and treat their specific emotional problems in terms of the meaning of the situation to the person and his particular personality. This can encompass a great deal of work, sometimes requiring intensive individual psychotherapy or psychoanalysis; couples or conjoint therapy; and/or intervention in family situations. The fortunate and reassuring outcome is that sizeable proportions of those so treated recover from their chronic disability and invalid state and are again able to function, justifying, I think, whatever effort it took.

The question now arises, "How does this individual experience compare to the general finding in present-day psychiatric practice?" One psychiatrist's experience may not reflect the experience of the field in general. A review of the current literature in the next chapter addresses that question.

4

Review of the Current Literature on Chronicity in Mood Disorders

The development in the last decade or so of the remarkably effective modern drugs for depression created a certain amount of overconfidence in medicines (psychopharmacology) and a tendency to minimize or even ignore psychosocial and psychotherapeutic methods and especially combined methods using all techniques. However, in the past few years workers in the field have learned that letting the family doctor prescribe even the most modern drugs and having the visiting nurse, or the pharmacist, or no one, follow the patient, does not cure people. The use of statistically accurate testing methods for medicines has been very helpful in identifying the drugs that are genuinely effective, as well as demonstrating in whose hands they are effective, and in whose hands ineffective. For example, a study by the Rand Corporation (Rogers et al. 1993) of a large number of patients with depressions showed that those treated by general practitioners and followed up after 2 years had much poorer results than a similar group treated by psychiatrists. It is now also apparent that even in the hands of psychiatrists—professionals trained in the use of modern medicines—the results leave much to be desired. No drug comes close to curing everyone.

Over the last few years, psychiatrists have accepted a number of concepts that address the problem of these patients who do not get well with medication alone. These concepts follow.

CONCEPT 1: CHRONICITY

Mood disorders are chronic illnesses and must be treated as such. Since the work of the Pittsburgh group was published, undeniably this concept has been the starting point of the new concepts (Kupfer 1997). This study demonstrated that rather than consider major depression simply as an acute illness, a new attitude had to be taken. Soon afterward, the new concept was clearly stated by Judd and his group (Judd et al. 1999): "There is increasing realization that unipolar major depressive disorder (MDD) is primarily a chronic disease with frequent episode relapses and recurrences across the life cycles and not merely an isolated single episodic illness." There is also an increasing recognition that residual subthreshold symptoms, i.e., "spectrum disorders," should be included in the group of mood disorders, as Judd and his group (1999) demonstrated.

Chronicity is not a transient impression but a fundamental enduring aspect of depression, as we know it. Kraepelin in his 1921 book made similar observations, specifically, that slight colorations of mood and the domain of personal predisposition represent the manifestation of a single morbid process. This recognition has made it necessary that we adapt our techniques to the concept of chronicity where indicated, not only in chronic cases but also in recurrent ones and those with residual symptoms—"spectrum disorders." The treatment techniques required are different from those techniques used for short-term cases and require special attention today, when, partly because of insurance considerations, short-term cases still are considered standard. The profession is now in the process of developing those techniques. Thase and Rush (1995) give a concise formulation of the problem.

The term *chronicity* currently refers to several overlapping clinical conditions that persist beyond and are related to the original mood disorder, as follows:

1. *Actual chronic persistence* of the original disorder under treatment. It is considered chronic if a patient who has received the appropriate and

currently available medications plus the standard attention to psychosocial problems does not respond with relief of symptoms.

2. *Spectrum disorders*, as described by Weissman (1999), refers to a watered-down version of the fully diagnosable disorder. Patients experience some relief of symptoms but residues of the original disorder persist enough to cause discomfort and disability. This response is more common than previously thought and is important in all the mood disorders, including unipolar and bipolar disorders.

3. *Subsyndromal Symptomatic Depression.* This disorder is very much like the spectrum disorders and also resembles dysthymia. It is defined somewhat specifically as "a depressive state with two or more symptoms of the same quality as in major depression excluding depressed mood and anhedonia. The symptoms must be present for more than 2 weeks and be associated with social dysfunction" (Sadek and Bona 2000, p. 30).

4. *Quality of life* (QOL) problems as represented in "insight, medication side effects, psychological distress, self-esteem, self-efficacy, coping, expressed emotion, and social support" (Ritsner et al. 2000).

46

Inasmuch as these phenomena have in common the property of chronicity, it is assumed that a predicament according to our definition will be present and can be detected by the method described in Chapter 5.

CONCEPT 2: TREATMENT RESISTANCE

Some patients do not respond well to medication. This concept followed quickly after concept 1 became widely acknowledged and accepted.

CONCEPT 3:
IDENTIFYING THE CAUSE
OF CHRONICITY IS IMPORTANT

Methods must be found that will identify early on the factors that make for chronicity and make it possible to treat these factors successfully. The symptomatic method of diagnosis used in this study—i.e., the Diagnostic and Statistical Manual (DSM-IV-TR™ (2000)—is very useful to identify and separate the different categories and symptoms. It makes possible aiming the therapy and identifying which therapy, which medication, which management will treat each symptom.

However, when a patient does not get well and becomes chronically ill because the standard treatment is insufficient, it is necessary to look at reasons and try to identify them. For example, what if the depression is useful in some ways, or if it is necessary for the patient to tolerate his life, or if it protects him in some way. For example, an article in the *Archives of General Psychiatry* is entitled "Is Depression an Adaptation?" (Nesse 2000). In summary, the author makes the point that the depression or low mood can be protective to the individual—protective against something worse. This idea is often held by society, family, loved ones, etc., who fail to recognize that it is also an illness with a great danger of suicide. Individual patients often need to look into any motives behind the low mood. This is one of the reasons for intensive psychotherapy in certain cases.

CONCEPT 4:
THERE IS A COMMON, UNDERLYING CORE PROCESS IN EACH CASE, WHICH SHOULD BE IDENTIFIED.

This important concept is not fully accepted but is beginning to receive greater recognition. As stated by Krueger (1999), after doing a factor analysis of comorbidity among mental disorders in a sample of 8,098 cases ranging from age 15 to 54 years, "comorbidity results from common underlying core psychological processes. The results therefore argue for focusing research on these core processes themselves rather than on their manifestations themselves." That is, don't focus just on symptoms, but on processes and causes.

CONCEPT 5:
BEYOND ACUTE SYMPTOMS, SPECTRUM DISORDERS, QUALITY OF LIFE, AND SEVERAL OTHER SYMPTOMATIC CLUSTERS

Aspects of the patient's functioning and quality of life (GAF and QOL) must be taken into account.

> There is increasing interest in assessments that capture a spectrum of outcomes beyond symptoms. Traditional depression scales assess the core biological features of the illness, mood, pessimism and vegetative signs (e.g., appetite and sleep loss). However, assessments of drive, motivation, performance, and quality of interpersonal relations (e.g., the social context once the symptoms are improved) may not be captured in the traditional symptom scales. [Weissman 1999]

CONCEPT 6:
THE DOCTOR-PATIENT RELATIONSHIP IS ESPECIALLY IMPORTANT IN CHRONIC MOOD DISORDERS AS A THERAPEUTIC DEVICE.

Outgoing APA (American Psychiatric Association) President Allan Tasman, M.D., urges

49

fellow psychiatrists to recommit themselves
to the "primacy of the doctor-patient relationship in psychiatric care." [*Psychiatric News*,
vol. 35, no. 12, June 16, 2000]

The doctor-patient relationship is important to:

1. Prevent suicide.

2. Give a patient who feels without value a sense
   of value and/or importance.

3. Allow working through and correction of long-
   standing problems.

CONCEPT 7:
COMORBIDITY IS OFTEN A CAUSE
OF TREATMENT RESISTANCE AND
DEMONSTRATES A CORE PROCESS.

Comorbidity refers to the coexistence of another factor, usually a diagnosable illness, that can influence
the treatment process. For example, the presence of a
physical illness such as heart disease or a psychiatric
illness such as an anxiety disorder that needs treatment can complicate and prolong the treatment of the
depression. There are other factors that can affect the
treatment process, such as old age. The geriatric
population differs from the general adult group in
response to medication and other treatments.

A concept not yet accepted by the profession has recently been formulated as a guiding principle, growing out of clinical comorbidity, as follows: When comorbidity occurs, such as "depression" and "anxiety," "these factors are most appropriately conceived of as 'subfactors' of a higher order internalizing factor" (Krueger 1999). Krueger concluded that "comorbidity results from common underlying core psychological processes. The results thereby argue for focusing research on these core processes themselves, rather than on their manifestations as separate disorders." However, others say that treatment must be directed toward the separate subfactors of the comorbid state, e.g., depression and anxiety (Wittchen et al. 1999). This book is directed toward identifying and treating a core process—the predicament.

In this book, I present and examine a number of cases of comorbidity treated by conventional methods, and then examine them and identify what might be considered a "higher-order internalizing factor." Symptomatically, some of them are better but functionally they are not well. In a number, there is a powerfully effective primary factor, which continues to operate and continues to produce symptoms that are secondary factors. Identifying a powerful primary factor and dealing with it can solve the problem of a chronic or refractory case and get the patient back into the mainstream of society. I call this primary factor a "predicament" that must be identified, as described in Chapter 5, and solved by treatment, as described in Chapters 6 and 7.

In summary, it appears that the recent literature is in agreement with my findings described in Chapter 3, namely, that a significant percentage, anywhere from 30 to 40 percent of patients, treated by psychiatrists, become chronic and many of these patients continue to respond only partially to current treatment methods. The pathway to chronicity is shown schematically in Figure 2. Some of these are relieved of symptoms but still do not function satisfactorily. It is to these groups that we now address our efforts.

Figure 2.   Pathway to chronicity in mood disorders.

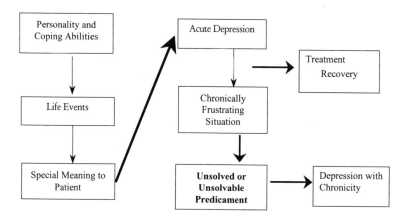

5

Identifying the Predicament Using the Multiaxial System of DSM-IV

Once the immediate pain is relieved, you may need to look at your situation and try to identify your predicament. There may be things you will want to change by means of counseling or psychotherapy. (Badal, 1988, p. 215)

The Multiaxial System of the *Diagnostic and Statistical Manual* (American Psychiatric Association 2000) has stood the test of time. The explanation of the details of the system in the manual (American Psychiatric Association 2000, pp. 27–36) is precise and useful. Application of the system can give a broad yet specific view of the patient's current problem as well as of the individual patient's life. The system seemed to me ideal as a measure of the problem contributing to the chronicity of the mood disorders I am focusing on in this study. Using the system, I have developed a method of measuring the predicament in order to compare patients with respect to difficulties in treatment. The method also may help to explain the chronicity and to illustrate and illuminate the specific characteristics that distinguish seriously chronic, difficult cases from those that respond relatively easily. This recognition should allow the physician in charge to focus on specific problems more efficiently.

The frequency of occurrence of chronic and refractory depressed patients is well established, and the presence of an underlying cause, a predicament that prevented recovery, was well documented. The question now arises, "How can we evaluate each patient and tell who is going to be chronic or refractory? Can it be done?"

In my original work (Badal 1979a and b) the predicament with two components seemed to be a large part of the cause of the depression. A principal component of that predicament was a very troublesome relationship with the important other—the mate or other most important person. A problem in the patient's personality made it impossible for the patient to control that relationship and solve the predicament. Thus the depression became chronic.

Since that study, a number of studies have reported on factors that could contribute to chronicity, such as comorbidity and poor response to medication. One helpful double-blind study showed that a combination of three variables predicted reoccurrence in 90 percent of cases of depression (Berlanga et al. 1999). The authors found that personality traits, treatment duration, and atypical response to treatment all influence the illness toward reoccurrence. Mazure et al. (2000) identify contributing factors to be stressful life events, previous history of depression, gender, age, genetics, and personality style. A number of other studies in the earlier literature are sources of factors contributing to recurrence and a chronic cause, including Klein et al. (2000), who thoroughly studied dysthymic disorder, concluding that it is a chronic condition with a protracted course and a high risk of relapse—almost all eventually develop superimposed major depressive disorder. Feske et al. (2000) note that anxiety is a clinically recognized correlate of poor outcome in the acute treatment of bipolar I disorder. History of panic attacks was a correlate of nonremission.

Berman et al. (1997) listed items that influence response, i.e., "clinical predictions of response" as:

1. Adequate dose. (Is the dose adequate?) Although this book does not delve deeply into the treatment with medication, it is important that the therapist know that some cases are chronic because of inadequate doses.

2. Adequate response. (How much symptomatology remains?)

3. Secondary to a general medical condition. (Often, results are complicated or prolonged by the medical condition.)

4. Secondary to a substance-induced mood disorder. (This complicates and prolongs results.)

5. Psychotic depression. (May often require more prolonged treatment, e.g., electroconvulsant treatment.)

6. Seasonal depression. (Sometimes a predictable source of resistance to treatment.)

7. Comorbid anxiety symptoms and panic disorder. (Both complicate treatment results.)

8. Bipolar depression. A mood disorder with very special needs, and potentially chronic in the same sense as Major Depressive Disorder.

9. Personality disturbances. (Often cause chronicity of mood disorders and require more intense psychotherapy, depending on type and severity.)

    a. Chronicity

    b. Severity

10. Early life stresses and current stressors. (Have to be taken into account as possible causes of resistance.)

These studies led me to update my previous structure of the predicament. I have added new factors rather than allowing the predicament to result from a combination of only the two components I originally observed and described in my earlier paper, i.e., (1) an unsatisfactory interpersonal relationship with the important other plus (2) a personality deficit that prevents the person from solving the relationship problem. I have added a number of other components derived from the later studies just described. Sixteen elements will be observed and graded on a basis of 0 (none) to 5 (seriously disabling) (Table 5-1). Then, to simplify the process, I have the therapist, after evaluating the patient on this detailed scale, continue to keep that preliminary score in mind when doing the next step, the really diagnostic step—the Multiaxial tabulation, on which the patient's final score and evaluation depends.

As to where you get the information identifying the elements that make up the predicament, don't expect the patient to tell you very specifically that the problem is his relationship with his spouse or long-time lover or others. You probably will have to read between the lines and ask questions to illuminate that point. He or she is just as likely or more likely to complain about symptoms. In fact, he may not have figured out that his depression may originate in frustration caused by a disturbance in his relationship with his important other.

As an example, in a review of a book subtitled "A personal account of one man's battle against chronic depression" Joyce Carol Oates (2001) gave a thorough and comprehensive critique of the author's subject,

Table 5–1. Factors contributing to chronicity of mood disorders (negative factors) and the scale used in scoring the factors.

Factor Number	Factor Description	Scoring Scale
1	Diagnosis, such as bipolar or schizoaffective psychosis	1–2 for schizoaffective or bipolar or cyclothymia
2	Severity of illness	5 for most severe
3	Neglect of treatment	5 for serious neglect; 0 for no neglect
4	Inadequate or incorrect medication	5 for serious inadequacy; 0 for no inadequacy
5	Poor response to medication	5 for very poor response
6	Need for medication	5 for required medication of the standard type; 0 for no need for medication
7	Judgmental defect	5 for longstanding defect
8	Personality deficit	5 for serious deficit interfering with function or interpersonal relationships

9	Family history	5 for strong history in the immediate family; 0 for no family history
10	Low level of family or other support	5 for no support; 0 for good support
11	Early loss or trauma, such as the death of the parent	5 for great; 0 for no early loss or trauma
12	Deficit in functioning	5 for no functions; 0 for no deficit
13	Comorbidity-psychological, such as depression plus anxiety	5 for great; 0 for none
14	Comorbidity-medical, such as a disabling disease	5 for great; 0 for none
15	Current loss or trauma due to illness	5 for serious; 0 for none
16	Current loss or trauma not due to illness	5 for serious; 0 for none

that is, a personal account of his chronic depression. The review showed that the patient who wrote the book did, indeed, fill the pages with vivid descriptions of his symptoms and yet did not point out the theme that a psychiatrist or therapist would have selected as the most likely to represent the "significant other," with whom he was having trouble enough to bring on a depression; and that was a part of the predicament he could not solve. A very brief but vivid description was given of an incident that revealed this most likely relationship, i.e., "—he began plotting murders in his mind," and assaulted a lover whom he suspected of betrayal. "I attacked him," he writes, "with a ferocity unlike any I had experienced before." So, I ask, he had a lover whom he cared about enough to do this? Isn't it likely that something very important in his love life was bothering him enough to be a serious factor in his depression? Yet he wrote a book of 571 pages about all kinds of symptoms with only a passing reference to the most important thing in a human being's life, that is, his love relations, the significant other, a most important thing in the lives of most people.

To simplify the scoring process, I put together two lists from observations available in the literature and clinical experience, one of factors occurring in the usual chronic, refractory, and treatment-resistant cases (Table 5-1) and another of factors that have been found to contribute to good recovery of normal functioning (Table 5-2) and transferred the recent observations from the literature to the Multiaxial System.

Table 5–2. Factors that act to mitigate chronicity (positive factors) and the scale used in scoring the factors.

Factor	Scoring Scale	Scale Transferred to DSM-IV
1. Strong character and a lack of character pathology	3–5	4–10
2. Good response to medication early on	4–5	4–8
3. Early psychotherapy, especially with insight	4–8	4–10
4. Strong support system	4–5	4–10
5. Positive interpersonal relationships	4–5	4–10
6. Current intensive psychotherapy	3–5	4–10

(The sum of scores transferred to DSM-IV was substracted from the sum total score of negative factors in Table 5–1 for the final score of each patient.)

In order to bring the original definition of the predicament up to date, the recent observations in the literature as to causes of chronicity and refractoriness should be evaluated. Table 5–1 lists those most valuable to add to the original 2 items. Sixteen items are listed, obviously including the 2 items named as the source of the predicament, i.e., (1) an intolerable relationship or environmental factor plus (2) a personality deficit preventing a solution of that problem. Table 5–3 shows approximately how these 16 factors relate to the Multiaxial System of DSM-IV and how

Table 5–3. Relation among the six categories in the DSM-IV Multiaxial System and the sixteen factors found in recent practice and literature to be important causes of chronicity.

(Factor numbers correspond to numbers in Table 5–1.)

DSM-IV Category	Factors	Description of Factors and Total Possible Points for Each
I. Diagnosis	1,2,6,7,13 (possibly 12)	Official name of illness and estimate of severity Need for medication Comorbidity (depending on severity) *Each can contribute up to 5 points toward the 10-point score.*
II. Personality Diagnosis	3,4,7,8 (possibly 12)	Neglect of treatment Incorrect medication due to noncompliance Serious judgmental defects Personality deficit *Each can contribute up to 5 points.*
III. Medical Issues	14	Evaluation in points depends on the severity and effect of the medical illness *Can contribute up to 10 points.*

| IV. Psychosocial and Environmental Problems | 9,10,11,12,16 | Family history
Prolonged grief and mourning
Low level or support
Early loss or trauma
Defect in functioning
Current loss or trauma
Each can contribute up to 5 points. |
| V. GAF (Global Assessment of Functioning) | 2,5,15
(possibly 7, 8) | *These can contribute up to 10 points each:*
Severity of illness
Poor response to medication
Current loss or trauma
These can contribute up to 3 points:
Neglect of treatment
Judgmental defect
Personality defect
For the purpose of scoring for diagnosis of chronicity, these are considered negative scores, whereas the GAF is typically given in positive numbers. |

they are used to compile the negative score. The positive factors that counteract the negative influences are listed in Table 5–2. They are subtracted from the negative score for the final score of each patient.

Using the Multiaxial System, I present a method to predict which patients will be refractory to the initial, ordinary methods of treatment and will need more intensive, more complex, long-term treatment, thus preventing the refractory course we see so often. This system can be applied at the outset or later on when the patient is better known and it becomes apparent that there are some long-term problems.

APPLICATION OF
THE MULTIAXIAL SYSTEM

In advance, be warned that the scoring system can be frustrating. Many will find it unnecessary actually to do the scoring once they have been alerted to the factors outlined in Tables 4 and 5 and described in the text. If these factors are borne in mind, it is likely that a knowledgeable and well-trained therapist will be able early on to spot those patients likely to become chronic.

Of the 9 issues highlighted under Axis IV in the *Diagnostic and Statistical Manual* (American Psychiatric Association 2000, pp. 31–32), those significant for the current group, i.e., contributing to chronicity, are listed in Table 5–1. This list of negative factors (those contributing to chronicity) was applied to each indi-

Table 5–4. Clinical groups determined from application of the proposed method to 33 patients.

Group Number	Score Range	Number of Patients (Total 33)	Clinical Condition
1	1–10	11	Normal functioning. Symptoms under control. Back in the mainstream. Most had extensive treatment.
2	10–20	14	Some symptomatic relief and able to perform independently but with serious functional symptoms in interpersonal relations or behavior. In need of a more intensive program and more time.
3	20–30+	8	Incapacitated symptomatically and functionally. In need of a new, intensive program and chronic treatment.

vidual patient. The list of positive factors (those that contribute to good recovery) (Table 5–2) was scored also:

1. The axes were scored on a scale of one to ten, to indicate degree of pathology, a score of 0 indicating absence of mental illness. A score of 10

Table 5–5. Scores of each of the 33 patients, with sum of factors contributing to chronicity and sum of factors mitigating chronicity (positive factors). Patients were grouped by score, with groups assigned as follows:

Group 1 = Score <0 to 15 (11 patients)
Group 2 = Scores 16–30 (14 patients)
Group 3 = Scores +>31 (8 patients)

Patient	Sum of Contributing Factors	Sum of Positive Factors	Score (Contributing Factors minus Positive Factors)	Group
1	30	9	21	2
2	43	15	28	2
3	27	20	7	1
4	51	16	35	3
5	18	25	-7	1
6	31	20	11	1
7	34	19	15	1
8	53	11	42	3
9	40	18	22	2
10	17	26	-9	1
11	51	13	34	3
12	43	22	21	2

13	31	23	8	1
14	42	19	23	2
15	41	15	26	2
16	29	16	13	1
17	45	17	28	2
18	44	17	27	2
19	31	16	15	1
20	48	10	38	3
21	52	16	36	3
22	33	11	22	2
23	38	10	28	2
24	33	12	21	2
25	41	6	35	3
26	48	8	40	3
27	58	1	57	3
28	23	21	2	1
29	40	18	22	2
30	40	17	23	2
31	28	22	6	1
32	40	22	18	2
33	17	20	-3	1

indicates severe illness. The numbers were then added for a measure of severity. The diagnostic method used was DSM-IV.

2. Five items of the patients' history and examination were evaluated, also on a scale of 1 to 10, to grade positive influences. There is some assumption in two of the items, but they are a part of the patients' experience with his illness and experimentally were used in the following way: The three items were scored, and then added for a total of positive factors.

3. Total of positive factors was subtracted from the total of negative factors, giving a number used as the patient's final score.

4. The final score is then used to classify the patient as to clinical condition, as shown in Table 5–4.

Before using the Multiaxial System for diagnosing personality disorders, it is necessary to be clear as to how to separate a personality disorder technically from a clinical disorder. Here is a clinical example of the problem in the case of a man who suffers from recurrent major depressive disorder:

This is a 48-year-old successful businessman, subject to recurrent major disabling depressions requiring potent antidepressants. He had finally, after 2 months, recovered enough on bupropion (Wellbutrin) to go back to work. However, he had so much trouble getting started every morning that it was almost noon before he could bring himself to interview clients. Methylphenidate (Ritalin) was started, and almost immediately, within a week, on a dose of 10 mg twice each morning, he was functioning very satisfactorily. He insisted that the brand-name product worked better than the generic (methylphenidate). He said, "Wellbutrin helps my depression, but Ritalin helps my drive, my ambition." This alerted me to reassess his personality, and I was startled to realize that he was really a passive, shy individual; not aggressive or particularly self-satisfied. His previous success had been due to his intellectual depth and his devotion, his honesty, and his knowledge of the law. Apparently, the Ritalin overcame the handicap of his rather passive personality and his shyness and got him going. Of course, a low-grade depressive can have similar symptoms, but in this case, it seemed expedient to treat the residual symptoms after the drug Wellbutrin had stopped the disabling depressive mood. A higher dose of bupropion would have increased the side effects intolerably. Was it dysthymia? I could not call it dysthymia officially because there was only the one symptom, a physiological one. However, there are occasionally depressed persons who, when treated medically, will have one symptom remaining. I prefer to call it a characterological symptom of the impulse-behavior deregulation group.

In applying the Multiaxial System to each patient, I have attempted to use the concepts listed below to grade the personality. For negative numbering, I have used numbers 0–10 in a negative score, with 0 being no disorder and 10 being a full-blown disorder. I have used positive scores of 1 to 10 to grade constructive attributes. "In the psychiatric classification system, an enduring pattern of thinking, feeling, and behavior is called a personality disorder if it causes personal distress or poor functioning" (Harvard Mental Health Letter 2000).

Alternatively, the definition of personality disorder has been expressed as follows: (1) cognitive-perceptual, (2) affective, and (3) impulse-behavior disregulation are the important personality dimensions that need treatment (Soloff 1998).

General diagnostic criteria for a personality disorder (American Psychiatric Association 2000, p. 287) are an enduring pattern of inner experiences and behavior that deviates markedly from the expectations of the individual's culture. This pattern is manifested in two or more of the following areas:

Cognition (i.e., ways of perceiving and interpreting self, other people, and events).

Affectivity (i.e., the range, intensity, lability, and appropriateness of emotional response. With depression, sadness, guilt, shame, etc.).

Interpersonal functioning.

Impulse control.

The enduring pattern is inflexible and pervasive across a broad range of personal and social situations.

The enduring pattern leads to clinically significant distress or impairment in social, occupational, or other important areas of functioning.

The pattern is stable and of long duration and its onset can be traced back at least to adolescence or early adulthood.

The enduring pattern is not better accounted for as a manifestation or consequence of another mental disorder.

The enduring pattern is not due to the direct physiological affects of a substance (e.g., a drug of abuse, a medication) or a general medical condition (e.g., head trauma).

It is sometimes not easy to separate the personality from the chronic, clinical disorder (e.g., from a depression or hypomanic attack), but for clinical purposes it can be very helpful and practical to use a separate personality diagnosis and treat that condition also. In the long run, the patient will be helped by this clinical strategy.

RESULTS OF THE APPLICATION
TO PATIENTS IN MY PRACTICE

The analysis of 32 patients from my practice using this method revealed three distinct groups (Table 5–4). Examples of patients from each group follow the table.

Examples of Cases Scoring 20 or Over

Case I: Score = 35

The patient was diagnosed with major depressive disorder, recurrent, with alcohol and drug addiction. She was a woman, age 56, divorced, both depressed and alcoholic, on Medicare, with suicidal depression. She was treated with the following medications: Trazodone 250 mg, Paxil 30 mg, Neurontin 100 mg, tid, and Navane for hypertension of 145/110. She is currently using alcohol periodically and has been a cocaine abuser. She is also agoraphobic.

Her childhood was traumatic. Her father and mother divorced. She says, "My mother hated me because I remind her of my father, and she gave me to my grandmother." Married at 16, divorced after 2 children of whom she gave up custody. "I was not a good mother. I thought they would be better off with someone else."

Phase I: She was admitted to the hospital to be detoxified of alcohol and is trying to stay sober. This is the beginning of phase I of treatment, to try stopping the comorbid disorder that is preventing phase II. It is necessary for the complete therapeutic process to go on to relieve symptoms to allow phase II (continuation) to proceed.

Phase II: A hopeful sign is that she has enough ability to look at the reality of alcoholism and say, "I've got to quit drinking," and even in the face of her boyfriend trying to get her drunk, she says, "I won't." What makes it possible is identification with the A.A. group and a gradual trusting relationship with a therapist. In addition, the medication relieves enough of the depression so that she does not need the alcohol as an antidepressant.

Of course, it is all too evident that the grief and pain of her childhood is still with her and she has never had the opportunity to mourn. Compare this to the cases in the group with scores of less than 10, all of which have had extensive psychotherapy and experienced the process of working through the early traumas as well as the current interpersonal relationships. Also, a very trusting relationship has developed with the psychiatrist.

CASE I

Score	Treatment Plan
AXIS I. Score 10. Major Depressive. Disorder, recurrent, alcoholism, drug addiction (cocaine), phobic (agoraphobia).	Refer to alcohol program for group support. Paxil 30 mg, Neurontin 100 mg (tid).
AXIS II. Score 7. Passive Dependent Personality.	Intensive psychotherapy with counseling, psychodynamic, behavioral, interpersonal.
AXIS III. Score 5. Hypertension.	Navane; close medical supervision.
AXIS IV. Score 10. Living alone in a subsidized apartment. On Medicaid. Friends are psychopaths. No family.	Involvement with Alcoholics Anonymous daily program. Therapy group at nearby hospital.
AXIS V. Score 10. Not able to work. Personal relationships poor.	Get VNA involved in home visits.
TOTAL NEGATIVE FACTORS: 47	
POSITIVE FACTORS	
Current psychotherapy. Score 3.	Continue. Develop an involved relationship. This is the basis of success. Be available.
Medical support. Score 9.	
TOTAL POSITIVE FACTORS: 12	
NET SCORE (NEGATIVE minus POSITIVE): 35	

PREDICAMENT: She has no mate. Plus a submissive passive personality. If the void can be filled by a strong patient-therapist relationship and a substitute family in Alcoholics Anonymous, she can recover. The therapy plan has to be fitted to the needs. The medication is adequate to control the symptoms of the Major Depression, but functioning and further recovery will depend on the therapeutic process added to the medication.

Case II: = 33

Diagnosis: major depressive disorder, recurrent, personality deficit.

A late-middle-aged woman, professional, separated from second husband. She is very successful in her work as an attorney. Her first husband died after a long illness, during which she supported the family by hard work in her profession. Her childhood was tragic. She came from a wealthy family, but she had little contact with her too-busy father, and her mother was incapacitated by depression. Her first depression was at age 14, with some persistence until she went to college. She was very successful in law school and in private practice.

Her first marriage was happy, with 2 children. They were somewhat neglected by her because of her devotion to work when her first husband became incapacitated and eventually died. Her grown children and her second husband (divorced) ignored her most of the time, as did her very busy father and her depressed mother. She turned back to her work but developed severe hypertension and a major depression to which she had a poor response to drugs initially, and was depressed for months.

Phase I: Poor response to drugs. A change in medication gave a better response but there was a delay in rehabilitation because of her sense of abandonment.

Phase II: Anger and antagonism surfaced toward her family. She attempts to work this through in psychotherapy, but a serious medical handicap due to hypertension and obesity prevent complete response. A need for support became evident and we now arrange for a group therapy and a more intensive psychotherapy program.

Phase III: Not able to enter this phase as yet.

This is an example of how even those in the "carriage trade" can become refractory if there were early childhood traumas, hereditary propensity to depression, intercurrent serious medical disability, and abandonment. This leaves a job for the psychiatrist, who is all she has left. Group therapy in addition will be started when she is ready.

CASE II

Score	Treatment Plan
AXIS I. Score 5. Major Depressive Disorder, recurrent.	Medication with antidepressants, etc., no letup, chronic dosage.
AXIS II. Score 9. Personality disorder—histrionic and narcissistic.	Intensive psychotherapy.

AXIS III. Score 10. Obesity, hypertension, out-of-control eating disorder.	Weight-loss program, monitored; intensive supervision.
AXIS IV. Score 10. Interpersonal relations poor. No support.	Family involvement. Group support. Development of long-term doctor-patient relationship.
AXIS V. Score 8. At Work. Scoare 8. In Personal Life.	Counseling needed. Counseling needed.
TOTAL NEGATIVE FACTORS: 50	
POSITIVE FACTORS	
Early psychotherapy. Score 3.	
Current psychotherapy. Score 5.	Continue with type of therapy. Personalized—interpersonal, psychodynamic, behavioral.
Medication response. Score 9.	
TOTAL POSITIVE FACTORS: 17	
NET SCORE (NEGATIVE minus POSITIVE): 33	

PREDICAMENT: She has no partner, neither a mate nor any supportive family member. Her personality is so narcissistic that she drives people away. Her illness really started in childhood, and she needs to solve this predicament by intensive therapeutic relationships to make up for the lack of supportive persons in her life. At her age, this is not easy. We will try to have her form a long-term, supportive relationship with a therapist and group relations that are supportive. Her medical condition has to be monitored closely also. A long period in a therapeutic setting such as a sanitarium may do as a start.

Case III: Score = 30

Ms. L., middle-aged single woman, a very successful commercial artist, earning $100,000 a year. Ms. L. is a handsome woman but dresses sloppily. She is very outgoing but sensitive to slights. Others at the firm find it hard to relate to her. She feels uncomfortable with her colleagues and they with her. Ms. L.'s talent is so great that they keep her on despite the handicaps.

She found herself struggling to understand why people find her difficult. At that time, she had classical major depression but it was mixed in with hypomanic features of overspending, sexual overstimulation, and affairs with inappropriate men.

Phase I: The depression only partially responded to medication. Later, she revealed that she was drinking most of a bottle of wine every day to put herself to sleep at night. As she cut down on the drinking, the antidepressant and the mood leveler worked better.

Her childhood was traumatic. Her father was a chronic depressed and alcoholic person. She became a loner, keeping away from people. Then, in her adolescence, she immersed herself in her painting, becoming a commercial artist. Her disability was not in her professional life but in her social relationships and her business judgment.

Phase II: Ms. L. is now beginning to work on her interpersonal relationships and her character flaw of lack of judgment financially. She is seen once a week to work on social relationships and issues of judgment.

Phase III: Not yet begun.

CASE III

Score	Treatment Plan
AXIS I. Score 10. Diagnosis, Bipolar 2, sometimes approaching Bipolar 1; alcohol dependency; alcohol abuse.	Giving up alcohol is primary; refer to alcohol program. Medication: verapamil 360 mg, Sonata 5 mg, #2/hs, lorazepam 0.5 mg Qid, Zyprexa 2.4 mg bid, Glucophage 1000 mg
AXIS II. Score 8. Personality disorder, not otherwise specified; very serious obstacle.	Intensive psychotherapy, preferably psychoanalysis later.
AXIS III. Score 5. Hypertension, diabetes.	Intensive medical supervision.
AXIS IV. Score 8. Serious interpersonal problems. Serious judgment problems with housing, money. Control problems. Little or no family support.	Psychotherapy and supervision, eventually psychoanalysis.
AXIS V. Score 8. Global assessment of functioning very low (3) except at work.	As under AXIS IV.
TOTAL NEGATIVE FACTORS: 42	
POSITIVE FACTORS	
Early psychotherapy: Score 0.	
Current psychotherapy. Score 6.	Continue. Develop an involved relationship. This is the basis of success. Be available.

Medical support. Score 8 or less.	
TOTAL POSITIVE FACTORS: 14	
NET SCORE (NEGATIVE minus POSITIVE): 28	
PREDICAMENT: Looks like a poor refractory outcome unless something very positive is done.	

Examples of Cases Scoring 0–10: No disability. Patients back in the mainstream in personal life and work.

Of the 9 cases scoring 10 or less, only 1 had a problem with alcohol or drugs and he had a questionable overuse of alcohol. All cases either had been or were in intensive therapy. One of the patients had a 5-year analysis previously, with good results.

Case IV: Score = 8

This case presents a married woman, aged 70, who was retired from her business. She was retired for 2 years by a heart attack, from which she was recovering slowly. She had been severely disabled by the heart attack and came back into once a week therapy because of anxiety and the necessity of adapting to an entirely new life style of physical invalidism.

She had two severe depressions early in her career. She was diagnosed with bipolar II, depressed phase. On medication for 30 years and with a 5-year classic psychoanalysis, she had a very successful career, had been able to be the main support of her family, always maintaining a marriage not entirely satisfactory because of husband's sexual problems. Now recovered back to social functioning on medication (Prozac and Depakote).

This case illustrates the successful use of medication plus intensive psychotherapy in a woman with a previous psychoanalysis. She has no serious disability at present. In the analysis, which was a classical analysis, 5 days a week, with a working through of a very traumatic childhood—a father who brought women into the house and was probably hypomanic, a mother who remained steadfast throughout. The family remained intact and did create a home with a mother and a father, providing a secure standard despite the father's adventures. Although the transference was analyzed, she remained in a somewhat flirtatious mood, transferred from the father, but controlled within the analysis. Thus, the analyst remained a father figure and a source of support and strength to her in her very demanding business, in which she was constantly and repeatedly flirted with and propositioned by clients. This is one of the results of psychoanalysis in persons who are needy because of the depressive tendency. Despite the analysis of the transference, the analyst also remains a real figure who is a friend in need and a parent substitute in the future. With patients who have suffered and could later be threatened by a return of their illness, the analyst can be turned to and should be available.

But, equally important in maintaining her stability and freedom from depression, her husband could now be an "important other," in his newfound assumption of a dominating and protective posture in the family. This is another patient for whom the support of an "important other" can provide a stabilizing force and keep the patient out of depression. The predicament of the patient is solved now because she has a stabilizing force in her husband, and her personality stability allows her to make realistic, sensible decisions in critical situations.

CASE IV

Score	Treatment Plan
AXIS I. Score 3. Diagnosis, Bipolar 2.	Medication: tricyclics and verapamil got good control. Changed to Prozac and Depakote because of side effects. Liquid form of Prozac because of allergy to dye in powder.
AXIS II. Score 3. Fairly normal personality.	Intensive psychotherapy, preferably psychoanalysis later.
AXIS III. Score 3. Allergic to some medications, but well-controlled on various medications.	Intensive medical supervision.

AXIS IV. Score 8. No dysfunction through adult life but has problem daughter and husband.	
AXIS V. Score 3.	
TOTAL NEGATIVE FACTORS: 20	
POSITIVE FACTORS	
Early psychotherapy: Score 10.	Classical psychoanalysis 5 days a week for over 5 years 25 years earlier.
Response to medication: Score 9.	
Functioning: Score 9.	Able to accept semi-invalidism after heart disease. Active social life. Let retired husband take charge. Accepted his impotence.
TOTAL POSITIVE FACTORS: 28	
NET SCORE (NEGATIVE minus POSITIVE): −8	
PREDICAMENT: The marriage was not perfect but her personality was able to handle it, by hard work, earning more than her husband but liking it. Thus, no predicament currently, as she solved the stressful relationship.	

Case V: Score = −1

Ms. J., a late-middle-aged widow with grown children, social worker in an inner-city agency, retired because of hypertension and heart disease. She had a very demanding job. Ms. J. was advised by her physician to retire. Although she performed the work effectively, the demands of the job endangered her and she elected to retire. Ms. J. had a normal social and personal life. Her interpersonal relationships are healthy.

Ms. J.'s childhood was normal, with no severe trauma. She was widowed in middle life, while her children were in adolescence. Ms. J. worked and brought up the children for 15 years by herself. Now that the children are grown, she has an active social life; she has dates and is active in her volunteer job. She is functioning as a person with normal life except for some limits caused by her hypertension.

CASE V

Score	Treatment Plan
AXIS I. Score 2. Diagnosis, mood disorder (depression), mild to moderate, due to medical illness.	Form good relationship. Counseling and intrapersonal psychotherapy.
AXIS II. Score 0. No significant pathology. Characteristically outgoing, responsible, reliable, affectionate.	Psychotherapy of counseling type when needed. Be available for advice.
AXIS III. Score 10. Hypertension, moderate. Moderately severe heart disease with limitations, but no failure. Enough to limit her work in a stressful environment with physical demands.	Make sure treatment is given by physician.

AXIS IV. Score 2. Interpersonal relations good. Environment good. Independent but modest income.	No intervention needed; she has good judgment.
AXIS V. Score Work 2, Personal 0. Global Assessment of Functioning 8. Some limits because of heart disease.	
TOTAL NEGATIVE FACTORS: 16	
POSITIVE FACTORS	
Early psychotherapy: Score 2.	Cooperative.
Current psychotherapy: Score 5.	Good judgment.
Response to medication: Score 10.	
TOTAL POSITIVE FACTORS: 17	
NET SCORE (NEGATIVE minus POSITIVE): −1	
PREDICAMENT: No predicament, by definition. The first half of the predicament is present, i.e., she has no mate and is looking for one. However, the second half of the formula making up the predicament is lacking, as she has no personality deficit and has strong personality factors. For example, she can form good relationships. Family support good to excellent. She has the ability to sublimate with volunteer work and good social relations.	

These stories illustrate how refractory cases can be identified if the Multiaxial system is used mathematically and the patient is scored on the basis of numbers. The completely recovered patients score 0–10, the functional but still somewhat symptomatic patients score around 10–20, and the refractory cases score 20 and above.

By identifying the elements contributing to the higher negative scores, it was possible to identify the 3 groups (Table 5–5), and with the elements of the Multiaxial system it is possible to tell which elements need to be treated and which positive elements are helpful for relief.

An experienced psychiatrist, seeing and interviewing a patient, will be mentally doing a great deal of this structuring silently and routinely, even without thinking of numerical evaluation, especially if he is oriented toward psychosocial factors and not merely making a symptomatic diagnosis. However, I think the Multiaxial Evaluation Report Form (DSM-IV-TR, p. 36) as given in the manual is sufficiently enriched by the information given with the numerical approach described in this chapter, that it becomes more usable as a way of planning treatment.

Part II will address the methods and process of treatment. Of course, the process of appropriate treatment for symptomatic relief is already in place, as the identification of the relationships and other important factors are identified and scored. The incorporation of all the factors into an evaluation of the patient gives the therapist preliminary insights as to the course of treatment. This is not simply a mechanical process of evaluation. Also, very importantly, a therapeutic relationship is being formed with the patient. The therapist, whether psychiatrist or other, is forming and growing empathy for the patient, and the patient senses that empathy and compassion. As the patient confides in the therapist and the therapist learns more about the patient, the patient feels that he is not with a stranger but a friend. With this in mind the process of therapy is already underway.

The fact that the therapist is working with a structured plan of action, i.e., the Multiaxial System, does not mean the patient contact has to be structured formally. It should be designed in such a way as to put the patient at ease and to start a relationship that will be effective in getting at the problem or problems that, hopefully, the patient will eventually be able to reveal and to grasp and understand.

The initial interview is important for several reasons. First, the patient may have some of the important issues immediately available for identification and recognition. Therefore, it is important that the therapist be able to listen carefully to what is brought up by the patient, whether spontaneously or in answer to questions. If the patient hints at something that could be very important, the therapist may want to hear more about it. Then, some of the forces at work will become clearer and will become part of the discussion.

This kind of understanding on the part of the therapist and his willingness to listen makes for a good therapist-patient relationship. Sometimes a depressed person finds it hard to talk, so the therapist has to be able to lead him or her into an opening up of whatever is on his mind, which he may never have faced or formulated. Perhaps he has only been dimly aware of, or even totally unaware or unconscious of the significance of the experience in connection with his depression.

I have found it useful, somewhere in the interview, to ask the patient to fill out the form of a very simple test, the Zung Self-Rating Depression Scale (Zung 1965). This test contains 20 significant items of symptoms that are to be checked off. This can be done in 5 minutes. They are worded in such a way as not to be upsetting to the patient. For example, "I feel hopeful about the future." There are four choices for an answer, namely, "none or a little of the time," "some of the time," "a good part of the time," or "most or all of the time." From the answers, the therapist can see just how hopeful or hopeless the patient feels, a very important piece of information in evaluation of how serious the depression is. With 20 such questions one can evaluate the actual intensity of the depression; and indeed, later can evaluate how the treatment is going and gauge the progress.

In this book, I have not explored the details of interviewing techniques, but the therapist, whether physician, psychiatrist, nurse, social worker, or psychologist, should be trained in working with people in distress. In so doing, an effective therapist-patient working relationship can be formed. The section on the doctor-patient relationship in Chapter 6 describes some of the general principles that have been found to work in these chronically depressed patients.

II

TREATMENT OF CHRONIC AND REFRACTORY MOOD DISORDERS

Introduction

The neurobiologist Erich Kandel (Kandel 1999a) suggested ways in which biology could influence the future of psychoanalysis. Some people took his theories to be a rejection of psychoanalysis. Later he wrote an answer to this impression: "I have great respect for the insight into human mental processes that psychoanalysis has opened up for us, and I believe that psychoanalysis provides the most coherent and interesting view of the human mind that we have" (Kandel 1999b).

So, does Kandel think the analyst's couch is obsolete? "No, absolutely not," he said. "Therapy has the potential, just as learning and memory do, to alter the brain's function at the gene level. And I think the methods of evaluating the outcomes, such as new imaging techniques, will provide indications of just that" (Kandel 2001, pp. 18–19).

In Part I, we verified the importance of chronicity and then described the techniques of identifying the predicament, which causes the chronicity and persistence of disability. These two chapters of Part II define and illustrate with case examples the treatment of the chronic and refractory cases of mood disorders via the predicament. Chapter 6 gives principles guiding the treatment, following the practice that in phases 1 and 2 the treatment is mainly directed toward symptom relief. In phase 3, the treatment is directed toward whatever *symptoms* are refractory to treatment in phases 1 and 2; plus the problem of malfunctioning, which may remain even when symptoms are controlled. Currently available treatment techniques are listed in Chapter 6. The ultimate goal in phase 3 is rehabilitation, making up for what was lost during the chronic years.

Examples of the actual treatment of *individual* chronic and refractory cases are in short supply in the recent literature. There is plenty of *statistical* information on certain specific limited techniques, for example, cognitive therapy, interpersonal therapy, and behavioral therapy, but the application to actual cases leaves something to be desired, namely, how to do it—how to combine medication with psychological techniques (and there are problems, even with those treatments that are statistically the most successful). The technique of individual therapy and its application needs more available descriptions. It is often necessary to use combined methods of psychotherapy, which uses combinations of counseling and interpersonal, behavioral, cognitive, and psychodynamic techniques. Why limit your therapy to one restrictive and limited technique if the problem is not limited? The components of the predicament will guide the methods of treatment.

One purpose of this book is to illustrate how one can use the weapons we have, how to apply what we have learned about the drugs, the psychosocial situation, and the psychotherapeutics; in short, how the battle is fought in the trenches. In Chapter 7, I will illustrate each type of the most difficult cases with examples—some successful, some failures. Although we have made and are still making substantial progress and have utilized some remarkably improved equipment and methods over the last decades, there are still serious problems to be solved with these most difficult cases. I will describe these patients and these difficulties and illustrate the techniques of combined therapy, aimed at the particular problems and personality deficits that constitute the predicament.

The discovery of many new antidepressants in the last decade has currently turned the attention of research in the mood disorders to these and even newer drugs and their chemistry. To some extent, this has had a narrowing effect on workers in the field as it diminished the attention paid to other important factors, especially the broader field of neurobiology, which is almost completely ignored by workers in clinical neurochemistry, who tend to focus on the particular receptor blocking of the particular drug.

There is great value in the neurochemistry known today. The particular receptor blocking and the effect of modern antidepressants on mood disorders are enormously important. However, research into more permanent changes by neurophysiologists shows that much broader issues are involved: for example, that abuse or neglect early in the life of an animal can cause permanent changes in the brain, which make it more susceptible to depression later in life (Nemeroff 1998). These changes apparently have been demonstrated in the human animal as well, i.e., that structural changes can be caused by a traumatic relationship with a parent (mainly mother and child.) The changes can persist into adult life and make the person more susceptible to maladaptive depressive symptoms into adult life. Note that this makes the adult respond more pathologically to stimuli and/or traumatic experiences than adults without that history (Schore 1994).

Chemicals do affect mood but more stable, long-term behavior and long-established patterns such as addictions, obsessions, compulsions, and phobias, which often are comorbid with depression, require something else also. Medicines are helpful in loosening the hold the obsession has but a new, overriding neural pattern has to be established as a replacement of the pathological neural pattern. This does not just happen with even the approved medicines. The same can be said for characterologic traits that are formed in early life. Long-term behavior patterns, consistent functioning, and the bases of interpersonal relationships, such as identifications, all depend on complex neural pathways and the stability or instability of these pathways. Individual chemicals expedite or block dominating pathways and networks, but they do not create these networks. This is where psychotherapy, environmental manipulations, occupational therapy, and psychoanalysis come in. Neurophysiologists have outlined the neuroanatomical networks involved in the development of behavioral systems in the brain, strongly influenced by childhood environmental stimuli. Neurochemistry can influence the networks; other pressures and reactors influence the long-term behavioral pathways also. This must be taken into account by anyone who treats mood disorders. Thus, combined drug and psychotherapies are becoming the accepted method, along with attention to psychosocial problems.

The availability of new and effective antidepressants and mood levelers has so occupied the attention of the recent generations of psychiatrists that intensive study of the various methods of psychotherapy has only recently been receiving adequate attention. In fact, learning the complex advances in psychopharmacology has become so demanding that there is too little room for intensive training in psychotherapy at the residency level. As a result, many psychiatrists trained in the use of the complex drugs available cannot do advanced psychotherapy and should use a trained psychotherapist for these more complex cases. Nowadays, this kind of "split treatment" is not uncommon (see Fawcett 2001).

"While residents are being trained to do a thorough diagnostic exam based on DSM-IV," Tasman

(2000) said, the next edition of the manual should incorporate provisions for "understanding the role of pathological conflict in developmental distress in the emergence of the symptoms we see."

Brief methods of psychotherapy are favored by today's researchers and motivated by today's financial pressures, although it would seem financially advantageous to find more successful methods. Nevertheless, so-called short-term cognitive therapy and, sometimes, interpersonal therapy are favored. The latter is derived from psychoanalytic principles, but psychodynamic therapy is generally not favored, at least not by name.

Over the last few years, definite evidence has been gathered that psychotherapy is effective, indeed sometimes necessary, and it has an important place in the treatment of mood disorders. The question is now open: "When, how, what method or methods?" What about psychodynamic therapy, since brief cognitive and interpersonal therapy, though often helpful, is far from the answer to everyone's problem. To look for the answer, we will now examine psychodynamic therapy and psychoanalysis as well as behavioral, cognitive, and interpersonal therapies. We start with psychodynamic methods.

In the decades before drugs were available, intensive treatment with psychoanalysis was shown to be helpful, even therapeutically successful in certain cases (Badal 1988). We will examine some of these cases to point out the areas in which psychodynamic psychotherapy or psychoanalysis can be helpful, often in combination with medication in patients with chronic mood disorders. The medications have opened up a field for psychotherapy in these cases by controlling the symptoms that concealed the patients' psychological personal problems. With the symptoms under control, the treatment can then focus on the patient's personal problem.

The chronicity of the illness in these cases has in many instances interfered with the patient's life so much that he or she is not in the mainstream and needs rehabilitation. The principles and cases of this rehabilitation are described in Chapter 7. Research and publications on psychotherapy for mood disorders in recent years has focused on time-limited and relatively brief methods of limited intensity, which we cannot expect to be successful with the more chronic and severe cases. This fact plus the emphasis on the available drugs, which reduce symptoms in almost two-thirds of patients, has made it easier to downplay psychotherapy, especially psychodynamic or any more intensive types. A recent remarkably objective and thorough study goes into this subject intensively and answers the question, "Is psychotherapy effective in the treatment of mood disorders?" (Thase et al. 2001). The title of the article is an indication of some of the doubts that have arisen in the profession and of course in the insurance industry—"Is Depression-Focused Psychotherapy Just an Elaborate Placebo?" The authors are very well-known experts in the field of quantitative front-line research in this field. They end the article with the statement (p. 60), "No! Depression-focused psychotherapy is not just an elaborate PBO (placebo)." They surveyed and combed the literature on five types of studies and came up with the following conclusions:

> "PBO (placebo based research) psychotherapy must be overseen by an expert to ensure that an allegiance effect does not influence outcomes."

> "Patients with severe recurrent or chronic depression may profit from a combination treatment of both psychotherapy and pharmacotherapy."

> "The use of psychotherapy after pharmacotherapy shows promise as a way to reduce vulnerability and improve long-term outcomes.

> "Depression-focused psychotherapy offers an ethical alternative to pharmacotherapy and is acceptable to a majority of patients seeking ambulatory treatment."

In the following chapters, 6 and 7, we explore clinical details of treatment, focusing on methods that are applicable to chronic and long-term difficult cases. We start where the summary by Thase et al. (2001) leaves off. The importance of the therapeutic alliance is explained and psychodynamic therapy is especially emphasized for its success in prevention. Psychoanalysis is described for its uncovering of long-range mechanisms, its clinical application in some cases, and very importantly, its use in understanding the predicament that has contributed to the chronicity of the patient's problem.

This section will focus on the treatment that needs to be done and allows for the circumstances in which it is done by one person—a physician who can both prescribe the medication and rehabilitation and the psychotherapy; or by two experts—one prescribing the medication and the other doing the psychotherapy, i.e., collaborative or "split" treatment (Fawcett 2001).

Advanced techniques of psychotherapy are required in many of these chronic cases. Many psychiatrists and physicians are not trained sufficiently to perform the sometimes complex interpersonal, developmental, and/or psychodynamic treatment required to be successful. As a result, the psychotherapy has to be done by a trained psychotherapist, while the M.D. continues to prescribe the drugs. This arrangement is known as "split treatment" and is becoming more common. It requires good communication between the two therapists, the medical and the psychological. An entire issue of *Psychiatric Annals* (vol. 31, no. 10, October 2001) is devoted to the problems and benefits of this method. Both psychopharmacologists and psychotherapists should read it.

6

Treatment Principles and Methods for Chronic Mood Disorders

GOALS AND PRINCIPLES OF TREATMENT

There is increasing interest in assessments that capture a spectrum of outcomes beyond symptoms. Traditional depression scales assess the core biological features of the illness—mood, pessimism, and vegetative signs, (e.g., appetite and sleep loss). However, assessments of drive, motivation, performance, and quality of interpersonal relations (e.g., the social context once the symptoms are improved) may not be captured in the traditional symptom scales. [Weissman 1999, p. 220]

A recent study by the National Depressive and Manic-Depressive Association (NDM-DA 2000) revealed that:

1. Most people depend almost exclusively on their family doctor for their diagnosis and treatment of depression. Seventy percent say they are satisfied with this situation.

2. Ninety-seven percent of doctors prescribe anti-depressants.

3. Fifty percent of patients say that medication controls their symptoms, but only 20 percent say it controls the symptoms completely.

4. Fifty-five percent of patients have stopped taking their medication at some time because of side effects.

Based on the study, the NDMDA recommended that doctors treating depressed patients talk to them more, explain the side effects of drugs more clearly, and adjust prescriptions more to accommodate individual needs.

The goals of treatment are both symptomatic and functional recovery. What do we mean by recovery? It is more and more agreed upon in up-to-date psychiatric circles that anywhere between 30 and 70 percent of patients with genuine mood disorders fall into one of these 3 groups—refractory, recurrent, or chronic. References with abstracts supporting this statement can be found in the reference section under Chapters 1 and 2. To this collection should be added a fourth group, referred to in Dr. Weissman's (1999) summary quoted above: namely, those who recover symptomatically as to basic symptoms on the diagnostic scale, but functionally do not recover satisfactorily in terms of drive, motivation, performance, and quality of interpersonal relationship. Because these 4 groups seem to be interrelated and interconnected clinically, I am directing the discussion in this book to all 4 groups. The case examples will, I hope, demonstrate the relations and interconnections.

The psychotherapist, medical or nonmedical, should also remember that when a patient or client with what looks like a purely psychological problem does not seem to be responding, he may belong to a group of mood disorders that are attenuated and will be able to do better psychotherapeutically with the help of medication (Freud 1971). This is yet another group of patients to be dealt with, a fifth group, which was described in the introduction as representative of the so-called *spectrum disorders*, i.e., not quite a complete illness but sharing some symptoms. They do not have the usual biological symptoms of anorexia, weight loss, insomnia, slowing down of thinking processes, and inability to function. That is the group of patients who really should not be considered biologically "ill" with an Axis I diagnosis but who are given medication by a busy physician. The medications we now have tend to be useful when a patient is worried about

something because the drugs such as Selective Serotonin Reuptake Inhibitors (SSRIs) make people feel
better sometimes without actually locating the real
problem and doing something about it. We will touch
on this group also.

Two principles must guide treatment of chronic
and refractory mood disorders. First, *the doctor-patient
relationship must apply* in the initial meeting and all
follow-up meetings. This principle refers to the sense
of responsibility on the part of the physician or other
professional dealing with the patient in trouble. The
relationship is evidenced by privacy, caring, taking
time, listening, and guiding. This is a primary therapeutic principle, with certain technical aspects, during
the treatment phases and the rehabilitation as needed.

Second, *the problem must be evaluated and re-
evaluated* by making a medical diagnosis, and finding
out how troubled the patient is and what is troubling
the patient in a personal way to whatever extent it
seems to be important. It is especially important to
evaluate for suicide—thoughts or plans—and if indicated, to take steps to protect the patient. Evaluation
also should include an initial estimate as to treatment,
and treatment should be started if appropriate. An
estimate should be made of how chronic the problem
is or will be. If enough details are available, an attempt
should be made to evaluate the potential for chronicity
by using the multiaxial technique described in Chapter
5. This may be difficult in the initial contact, and it
may have to wait until you know the patient better.

INDIVIDUAL TREATMENT TECHNIQUES

The Doctor-Patient Relationship

Special Developments in the Long-Term Relationship

Usually, chronic patients have to be under treatment for several years, and sometimes indefinitely, as in any chronic illness. However, in psychiatric illnesses particularly during this time, so much of the nature of the patient's life can influence the illness that the psychiatrist is given a great deal of confidential and intimate information that generally would not enter into the management and treatment of other chronic illnesses or of a brief psychiatric illness. What develops in the long-term physician-patient relationship is a special *therapeutic alliance* with certain special characteristics:

1. Dependency

2. Attachment

3. Transference.

A discussion of the interaction of these phenomena follows.

Dependency is realistic and convenient because the physician has accumulated all the information about the treatment and response of the patient over a long period and up to date. With that accumulated information, the psychiatrist is in a position to be knowledgeable, reliable, and available when needed. Of course, the nature of this dependency will also be influenced by the patient's personality, the nature of his interpersonal relationships, and his childhood training and experience. The reality is that if the physician is good and reliable, the patient can realistically expect him to know his business and care about doing it correctly. The doctor and patient have a common goal, interests, and dedication—to get the patient well.

Attachment, on the other hand, takes our appraisal of the physician-patient relationship in a direction that involves more than the realistic goal. It brings into the relationship some of the style of the patient's attachments that he or she has had all his or her life, learned in childhood. Bowlby (1969) described the development of the normal attachment in the human animal in childhood as a need for comfort and support and wrote that the model learned as a child will govern relationships of the adult. When sick, the chronic patient may revert to that relationship and become very dependent. The patient also may be very cooperative and successful in the treatment if the physician shows concern, interest, and support; and in that sense is comforting, especially to a patient who does not have very much self-esteem. In an article entitled "Attachment and the Therapeutic Relationship," Miller (2001) reports on a study by Ciechanowski et al. (2001)

that revealed that the attachment style of the diabetic patient learned in childhood had an important influence on the outcome of the therapeutic relationship in the treatment of diabetes in adult life. The adult diabetic who did not do well had especially experienced rejection as a child. Because we know that many adult depressives had traumatic experiences, losses, and rejections, we can assume that they will bring to the therapeutic relationship a style of attachment that will require a great deal of comfort and support as compensation before they can become independent.

Transference develops in long-term relationships where the position of the physician as the personal long-term authority puts him in a position to seem to assume some of the characteristics of the parent. If the patient feels that he has a parent substitute who regards him as important and supports him and clearly wants him to get well and be comfortable, the patient will respond positively because he wants to please the physician. If he thinks the physician doesn't care, he will have less motive for getting well. Transference is very complex and should be studied thoroughly in reference to the relationship (Greenson 1967).

A successful doctor-patient relationship requires that the doctor adopt the right emotional stance. An appropriate amount of concern, interest, support, yet with a sufficient degree of realistic optimism to balance the usual pessimism of the patient, is critical to developing a good doctor-patient relationship. The doctor must show a regard for the patient as worthy of attention to balance the usual feeling of depressed people as being unworthy. The doctor must also know when to intervene and when not to intervene. With long-term cases where there are character and personality problems that have to be worked through, a transference will develop that can be analyzed as an important part of the recovery and maturation process. The long-term case described in the chapter on treatment is a good example of how important this can be over and above simply giving medication to one of these more chronic patients. The relationship may actually become a reality, helping realistically with parental qualities. This may allow the patient to catch up on what he missed in childhood developmental phases.

The Therapeutic Alliance

Availability during periods of anxiety is especially important in the long-term doctor-patient relationship, for two reasons. First, it brings comfort, which is needed to bring about the kind of transference that opens the door to insight. Second, it gives the therapist a chance to understand and communicate to the patient insight into the cause of anxiety, the kind of insight that is the basis of successful treatment and ultimate cure.

Two examples are seen in the following cases. A very bright man of late middle age had been treated with considerable success for several years for phobias he had had since adolescence. Upon the therapist's retirement, the patient was referred to a very competent, experienced psychiatrist. A few months later, he found himself having trouble reaching the new therapist when a typical acute occasion arose when he needed comfort, relief, and insight. He said that he had decided to go to another new therapist instead of the present one because the new therapist was always available and always called him back when he left a message. Availability, availability, is the key to success. These chronic, long-term cases require techniques and insights that allow the patient to overcome a well-established symptom cluster, and the therapist has to be there to supply what is needed.

A second example is the case of a single woman, very bright, who was under the care of a psychiatrist for over 15 years, years marked by numerous admissions to the hospital for suicidal threats and episodes. The doctor-patient relationship continued through the ups and downs of her disease, which was not obviously bipolar and nowadays would be called bipolar spectrum. Numerous medications were tried, and she was kept going at a very low level. Then Prozac came along and it was tried, successfully. For the first time in years, she was able to function at her high intellectual level, and she was able to enter a rehabilitation program, go to graduate school, and work at a professional level. The therapeutic relationship had persisted all those years, with loyalty to the cause by both the psychiatrist and the patient. The doctor had always been there for the patient, had not committed her legally, had relied on her willingness to enter the hospital when he thought it necessary, and thus they had worked together over the many years, trusting each other—a true therapeutic alliance.

Techniques in the Doctor-Patient Relationship

For a description of the techniques involved in a successful doctor-patient relationship, the classic book by Brian Bird (first published in 1955; an enlarged edition was brought out in 1973) speaks with considerable wisdom. In his preface, Dr. Bird (1973) speaks of how people who have "discovered" his book wrote him about it and had "caught hold, not only of the *treatment issues* involved in talking, but of the principles which, when understood, contribute enormously to the usefulness of talking." Also in his preface, he writes about the "changing medical scene" (p. vi)—i.e., increasingly "elegant" drugs, computers, new ways of financing, privacy, and individuality. It is remarkably like the medical scene today. He stresses focusing on the "meaning behind the words," the importance of the patient, "not on what he says, but on what he actually thinks, feels, fears, and desires" (Bird 1973, p. vii).

Bird was a practicing and teaching (training) psychoanalyst, not an amateur philosophizer. He knew about talking to patients on a professional level. To answer the question "Are there techniques to the doctor-patient relationship?" read Dr. Bird's *Talking with Patients*. A study of this field especially will help recognize the underlying main human problems troubling the patient, whether or not he is aware of it.

Bird (1973, Part 1, pp. 1–254) devotes a special chapter to matters of concern to psychiatry and to mood disorders such as: the anxious patient, the angry patient, hidden anger, the overly affectionate patient, the crying patient, the bereaved, the guilty, the dying, the alcoholic, the depressed and suicidal, mentally ill, and affective response to surgery (lethargy, apathy, anger, depression, loss, etc.). Specific technical recommendations he makes are to give the session enough time; to create quiet, seclusion, and privacy; to allow few, if any, interruptions; to be cheerful, sincerely interested, and understanding; to use your eyes to look for signs of feeling; to be able to listen and avoid writing; to not hurry; to follow up what the patient says; and to be a "doctor"—display a personal sense of involvement and responsibility. *What begins to emerge in the doctor-patient relationship is an awareness of a particular need in the patient who has a clinical depression—a need to have a helpful someone whose role is support, understanding, availability; who also can provide the appropriate technical treatment, methods, and materials.* This role is reminiscent of Bowlby's (1969) description of the fundamental importance of a person to whom the human is attached and from whom he gets comfort and support (Miller 2001).

113

PHARMACOTHERAPY

The therapist, family doctor, and psychiatrist should know some general facts about the present-day discoveries, and by recognizing the complexity of the field be able to spot when a consultation is needed. It has been demonstrated that there is an enormous superiority in positive results of treatment in the hands of psychiatrists over the results with the family physician. A summary of the important insights of the current workers in this field was recently given by Delgado (2000) (2001).

Delgado emphasized that specific neurotransmitters selectively modulate different aspects of behavior. That is, the set of depressive symptoms resulting from a depletion of serotonin is different from those resulting from a depletion of norepinephrine. Also, drugs that affect multiple neurotransmitters may have a broader profile. Some of the more recent drugs do this, and are better tolerated than the older drugs. One clinical technique that works in supplying medication that affects multiple neurotransmitters has been to use 2 or more antidepressants of different classes. For more details see Delgado (2000) (2001) to understand how and why this works. Practicing psychiatrists and therapist who want to give the best treatment to their patients should read the details in this article to keep up with the latest discoveries.

Drugs have made it possible to overcome by psychotherapy some of the symptoms we now consider to be characterologic. In the future we can probably expect that even more of these personality traits can be treated efficiently by medication with even newer drugs.

This book will not deal with the details of pharmacotherapy, which would require an extensive discussion. Appendix I is a list of currently available medications used to treat mood disorders. The therapist can help by spotting problems of medication. If the therapist is a nonmedical therapist, he or she should report any problems to the M.D. who is prescribing the medication. References at the back of the book will lead the reader to detailed discussions of this type of treatment. The case histories provide examples of current drugs and methods.

PSYCHOTHERAPY—MANAGEMENT AND COUNSELING

A patient writes in the *New Yorker*, in typical *New Yorker* language:

> What do we think about psychotherapy? I don't mean for inpatients. They clearly need it; their lives are wrecked. I mean outpatients. The walking wounded among us. . . . For patients in serious distress, pills are useful, but they cannot provide, don't aim to provide, what psychodynamic therapy has at its core." (Acocella 2000)

The research of the last 5 or 10 years has clearly demonstrated that the combination of psychotherapy and medication outperforms others alone. Even the few diehards in the psychopharmacological field who had insisted for years that medication would do everything generally accept this. There are patients who can be controlled by psychotherapy alone. If you accept that psychotherapy is beneficial, then the questions become: What kind of psychotherapy and how much? The tendency in research has been to test individual specific treatments. Of course, any practitioner of experience and training knows that you fit the treatment type to the patient and that usually it takes a combination of types to do the job. As to how much therapy, one hopes that the practitioner does the amount that each job requires, despite insurance restrictions.

Researchers in psychotherapeutic methods in the last 10 years have tried to keep the methods tested pure and separate in the interest of statistical evaluation, e.g., cognitive is tested as purely "idea" therapy, which avoids feelings and tries to be strictly a technique for changing the patient's depressing and depressive ideas. Behavior therapy attempts to get the patient to behave in such a way that he will feel less depressed. Interpersonal therapy attempts to change the patient's important relationships by discussing how he or she reacts with others, especially the important others. The researcher typically tries to divide a group into 3 sections—one with a medication alone, one with psychotherapy alone, and one with both combined. Most research in the last decade in this area has demonstrated that the combined therapy works best, especially when interpersonal therapy is combined with a medication. Experienced psychotherapists, trained in several types of therapy, especially those trained in psychodynamic therapy—e.g., psychoanalysis—usually tailor the treatment to the situation.

So in this chapter, we start with psychotherapy in general first; then develop the psychodynamic method and give examples. We cannot go deeply into all of the specific varieties used by certain followers, such as cognitive behavioral therapy (CBT). The psychotherapist who understands the psychodynamic picture will have an understanding of the basis of the chronicity of these long-range problems.

Someone has to be in charge of the whole treatment program and to make decisions about the technical issues that arise along the way even though others may be involved. The patient has to know that he or she can consult the person in charge on decisions about the treatment and matters that have a bearing on it. That accessible person may also be providing the therapy in general, and the medication. If a psychiatrist is simply giving medication and not doing the psychotherapy, one of the pair has to know enough about what is going on in a complex program to make decisions about changes. This is an especially important role with the chronic, refractory, and often complex cases.

There are times with these illnesses that the person in charge has to step in and make a decision, such as when to hospitalize the patient or when to change the medication, to agree or disagree with some wish of the patient, or to present a plan. This is called counseling and is an important tool in the armamentarium of the psychiatrist. Even in intensive therapy such as psychoanalysis, when the counsel of the psychiatrist is needed, it is important that it be expressed to the patient and/or the family. The impact on the patient of the analyst doing more than analysis will have to be discussed as to its effect on the patient. Sometimes in analysis it works better to have someone else give the medication so that the analyst can retain his uncomplicated role, but in many cases the analyst can prescribe medication if a patient in analysis needs it.

The predicament underlines and emphasizes the importance of personality in creating the problem of chronicity. Therefore methods must be employed that solve the problem of personality characteristics that have prevented the person from solving or dealing with whatever of the problems has created the depressed mood. Methods must be tailored to the individual character problem feeding into the predicament. In both short- and long-term cases, certain of the problems seen in the patients with chronic depression are best solved by a process of analysis of the character problem that has prevented the patients from dealing successfully with the stressor causing the depression. For example, problems created by childhood experiences of the sort that caused excessive guilt, passivity, grief, anger turned inward, etc. In some cases, psychodynamic psychotherapy will work very effectively. In

118

others, a more thorough and penetrating working through will be necessary to eradicate long-standing and thoroughly imbedded characteristics. Examples will be given of each type in this section. Also see Berlanga (1999).

One problem may be lack of insight into what is really going on and contributing to the depression. When a personality that actually is fairly healthy does not consciously see the problem of the relationship, psychotherapy with interpersonal analysis may bring it to conscious awareness and understanding and the patient can then act to better the situation.

COGNITIVE THERAPY

An example of the use of cognitive therapy is the case of a middle-aged divorced, successful, very bright storekeeper who came for therapy because he thought he had Maladie des Tic (Tourette's Syndrome). All his adult life he had been self-conscious about his face, having had severe acne as an adolescent. I looked at him and said, "You can't have that. You don't have the disease." I assured him that speaking as a neurologist, which I had been, he did not have that disease. He jumped up and was very relieved to hear that it would not dominate the subsequent course of his life. However, that insight opened up to analysis the childhood and adolescent experiences behind the self-consciousness, and his therapy was able to progress.

119

That one "cognition" had blocked access to the traumatic experiences of his childhood that were the basis of his anxiety. Cognition therapy may in some cases be regarded as "idea therapy," even in one complex modern form described by McCullough (2000). Another combined form is cognitive behavioral therapy (CBT).

INTRAPSYCHIC THERAPY

Intrapsychic phenomena important to normal functioning can be absent or reduced when modern drugs are effective in reducing symptoms, as Weissman et al. (1974, 1997, 1999) have observed. Intrapsychic phenomena are treatable in the currently used cognitive, interpersonal, or behavioral treatments, which work well in certain cases; but can fail to alter some of the more deep-seated pathology, which can persist in some patients even with the use of any or all of these methods. Psychoanalysis and/or the psychodynamic method, on the other hand, can effectively modify long-standing fixations that persist from childhood on and have diminished the person's functioning as an adult in the mainstream of society.

PSYCHOANALYSIS AND ITS DERIVATIVES

The process of reconstruction (in psychoanalysis) integrates and transcends memory, facilitating personality reorganizations. [Blum 1999, p. 1125]

I now turn to psychoanalysis and its derivative, psychodynamic psychotherapy. In my experience, it has great value with these refractory cases and even more now that medication is available to enable more people to be psychoanalyzed. Current standard therapies, short term and limited, give statistical advantages to cognitive and interpersonal therapies, the latter a derivative of psychoanalysis. However, the statistics, though positive, are not very impressive and leave in their trail a great many cases that become chronic and refractory. The time seems appropriate to examine other techniques of psychotherapy that work on long-standing pathological personality problems. For example, psychoanalysis and psychodynamic therapy need more emphasis, particularly in cases with early losses that influence the child's development and set the groundwork for depression in adult life, which is a very common finding in refractory and chronic cases.

The predicament, as we have identified it, emphasizes the importance of personality in creating the problem of chronicity. Therefore, methods must be employed that solve the problem of personality deficits or characteristics that have prevented the person from solving or dealing with whatever problems have created the depressed mood. Methods must be tailored to the individual character problem feeding into the predicament. In both short- and long-term cases, certain of the problems seen in the patients with chronic depression are best solved by a process of analysis of the character problem that has prevented the patient from dealing successfully with the stressor causing the depression. For example, problems created by childhood experiences of the sort that caused excessive guilt, passivity, grief, anger turned inward, or unresolved grief (Badal 2000). In some cases, psychodynamic psychotherapy will work very effectively. In others, a more thorough and penetrating working through will be necessary to eradicate long-standing and thoroughly embedded characteristics. Examples will be given of each type in this section (see Berlanga 1999 and Angst 1992).

A psychotherapeutic method has been recently described that in effectiveness outdoes any on the market. Instead of obtaining positive results in 50 to 75 percent of patients, this method gets 95 percent improvement when given combined with medication. However, there is a catch to it. For one, the patients are highly medicated. Most important, this therapy is more intensive than most, starting with two sessions a week. It is also a combination of several types of techniques—cognitive, behavioral, and analytic.

This type of psychotherapy was called by its inventor "Cognitive-Behavioral Analysis System" (CBAS) (McCullough 2000), and was described as a modification of *interpersonal therapy*, in which the interpersonal relationships important to the patient were taken apart in a sense and their mechanisms verbalized, including the relationship with the therapist. In short, a method that would take into account what I have called the "predicament" involving a problem in the relationship to the "important other." A very important point of the technique was the frequency of the therapeutic sessions—2 sessions a week for 8 to 10 weeks, then 1 session a week for several weeks. This much intensity makes for a strong and emotional involvement on the part of the patient. In this respect, it has some of the intensity and involvement of psychoanalysis, although for a shorter time, and resembles the combined technique used by most experienced therapists.

In describing this method, McCullough (2000, pp. 17, 247) additionally discusses and names transference, a psychoanalytic concept that is also analyzed during the therapy, similar to the analysis of transference in conventional psychoanalysis. This method reads like a shortened psychoanalysis and combines psychodynamic, interpersonal, and cognitive methods, very much as the analyst does in a psychodynamic therapy. The title with 3 types named—cognitive, behavioral, and analysis—could easily add a fourth (i.e., interpersonal) and would be what I advise for refractory depressions.

Actually, it can be very helpful in psychotherapy, under any name, for the therapist to discuss and interpret some of the patient's ideas and attitudes toward the therapist as transference, especially when they seem to get in the way of insight on the part of the patient, or when the patient is carried away by the feelings. As pointed out by Tasman, quoted at the head of the introduction, the doctor-patient relationship is vital in these long-term, more complex cases, and to be able to analyze it (as well as to exploit it) can add an important developmental dimension to the therapy.

Especially where there is some developmental arrest—
say in a patient whose illness started in adolescence—
the transference can be used to good effect. Transference
works both ways, including the therapist's posture
vis-à-vis the patient, i.e., a very positive and interested
attitude puts him or her in the position of a good
parent who encourages gratitude and maturation.

Transference analysis in this type of therapy is
different from that in psychoanalysis and psychodynamic therapy derived from psychoanalysis. In Mc-
Cullough's method, which he calls "proactive," the
therapist actively points out that the patient's symptomatic behavior is derived from his earlier relationships and that it is different from the healthier way the
therapist treats the patient. The therapist uses this as a
method of obtaining a healthy, supportive relationship
with the patient to get the patient to feel encouraged to
discard the pathological aspects of his training that he
learned in his upbringing by contrasting them with the
way his therapist regards and treats him. This is an
active, structured therapy with almost everything done
at a certain time, unlike the usual psychotherapy in
which what comes up from the patient more or less
spontaneously will be at the center of interest. This
method requires fairly intensive training to learn the
steps, the timing, and the course of the therapy, and
would have to be learned in an authorized teaching
course. Actually, it seems that by showing actively how
considerately the therapist treats the patient in contrast to how his parents treated him is really a modified form of guidance and cognitive therapy, no matter

how successful it may be. Of course, it would help the patient to understand himself better and to feel better about himself when the therapist treats him with respect and does not criticize him.

Concerning the patient's reactions, McCullough states (2000, p. 103), "they learn to perceive that a new interpersonal reality exists between themselves and the clinician." Also, (p. 103), "The ideal outcome for both therapy systems is to demonstrate the obsoleteness and destructiveness of these negative interpersonal expectations and to replace them with new interpersonal perspectives." Of course, this further illustrates the importance of the patient-physician relationship, as we have emphasized. However, like so many of the short-term therapies, it emphasizes symptoms rather than causes, by treating "interpersonal expectation" as symptoms. I would expect that the long-term outcome would not be as good as the short-term.

McCullough's method also resembles psychodynamic psychotherapy in that it analyzes the interpersonal relationships that are heavily involved in the patient's life. Note that it is not called cognitive behavioral *therapy* but Cognitive Behavioral *Analysis* System, meaning that the mechanism was analyzed and not just named, i.e., a process of conventional psychoanalysis was used to help understand the symptoms. As we have learned, certain stresses and personal situations have fed into the patient's predicament and have led to chronicity. An important stress is problems in interpersonal relationships, so it follows that a

125

therapy that corrects the problem will relieve whatever stress the relationship is causing. This is particularly important as it contributes to the very predicament that caused chronicity in that patient. Apparently, what differentiates this system of psychotherapy from other, more short-term behavioral and cognitive systems is its use of psychoanalytic and psychodynamic principles and methods, analysis of transference, and more frequent sessions.

However, more than one area of the depressive's life feeds into the depression (for example, childhood trauma, which contributes to the personality problem of the predicament). So it stands to reason that if you can correct the influences of the childhood trauma, you can eliminate another potentially powerful depressogenic influence. That task is found in psychoanalytic psychotherapy alone of the methods. So if all other therapies deal with the immediate problem, e.g., an interpersonal one, someone has to find a solution to those that are "intra" personal. Psychodynamic therapy fills that niche.

COMBINED TREATMENT TECHNIQUES

The introduction of effective medications for depressions and for bipolar diseases has opened up a new field for psychotherapy, i.e., persons under treatment with antidepressants who originally were too sick to deal psychotherapeutically with their personal and

personality problems. The following letter from Anna
Freud illustrates the point:

> As far as I am concerned, I have had great
> help from medical colleagues used to the
> administering of modern drugs, with three
> patients in severe states of depression. In all
> of these cases, the therapeutic use of drugs
> did not in any way interfere with the progress
> of the analysis, quite on the contrary, it helped
> the analysis to maintain itself during phases
> when otherwise the patient might have had to
> be hospitalized. Only in one of these cases
> some difficulty was created for a short time
> by a somewhat excessive drug prescription,
> which made me feel suddenly that the patient
> ceased to be himself.
>   I think I would feel very different if drugs
> were used to bring material with which the
> patient found it difficult to deal. In cases like
> that the situation would be rather near to that
> of hypnotized patients whose resistances are
> overrun by an external force instead of being
> worked through gradually. [Freud 1971]

Loeb and Loeb (1987) report how several bipolar
patients undergoing psychoanalysis were able to identify an oncoming manic attack early and increase the
lithium dosage enough to avert the attack.

Among researchers and the younger generation of
psychiatrists, especially those who write and publish,

the function of psychotherapy in the treatment of mood disorders was relegated to an almost negligible role for years after a host of effective antidepressant and mood-regulating drugs came on the scene. For years, there had been a polarization among clinicians until it became evident that pharmacotherapy is indeed very effective but that in many cases something else is needed. Likewise, in the last few years it has become increasingly evident that some forms of psychotherapy can improve the results in the treatment of patients with mood disorders. This improvement is due to the specificity of psychotherapy for problems not solved by drugs.

For example, dysthymia is a chronic form of depression sometimes present since childhood, similar to what was called depressive neurosis in earlier editions of the *Diagnostic Manual*. In a recent study of dysthymia, Haykal and Akiskal (1999) said, "We therefore suggest that, until proven otherwise, psychotherapy in dysthymia be used as an adjunct to pharmacotherapy. Nonetheless, as the vignettes we present attest to, the long-term management of dysthymia with pharmacotherapy is an art that requires not only broad clinical experience in pharmacotherapy, but also a thorough understanding of the *interpersonal context of depression.*" This implies that the long-term treatment of depressions requires a relationship with a therapist who will understand the patient's interpersonal relationships and help the patient solve the problems of those relationships, by some form of psychotherapy. In previous articles, the authors had said that any psychodynamic psychotherapy was in-effective—a very narrow and limited attitude. There is of course much importance in the *interpersonal* psychology, which usually also involves the *intrapersonal*, which consists of certain values and mechanisms behind the problems that led into the illness. Ignoring the interpersonal psychology also leaves out of the treatment the meaning of the interpersonal problem and its basis, which may require a psychodynamic approach to be helpful, and of course, that may sometimes require analysis of the transference relationship with the physician. We are speaking here of the chronic cases that have not responded to the simpler methods described by Haykal and Akiskal (1999) described above. It will be interesting to see if the high level of positive response to the techniques of McCullough (2000) holds up with time. It has the elements of a psychodynamic method, with its analy- sis of transference, more frequent visits, and other characteristics, such as working through memories of childhood traumas by transference analysis.

Recent research findings (Fenton 1997) convinc-ingly demonstrate that a flexible form of individual psychotherapy, when combined with appropriate neu-roleptic medication, can yield improvements in social and vocational functioning unobtainable with "treat-ments as usual." "People are saying, 'I want my doctor to spend more time with me,' says Dr. David Stern [Stroh 1999], an assistant professor at the University of Michigan Medical School."

Fenton's article describes the evolution of the use of psychotherapy in schizophrenia, which nowadays has increasingly taken an effective role in the illness. He describes a therapy called *Personal Therapy*, a flexible form of therapy combining a variety of techniques applied flexibly and based on the individual's phase of illness and type of illness. This description could be applied also to the most effective psychotherapy for mood disorders. This technique is in contrast to the reports in the literature of the application of strictly limited forms of psychotherapy—cognitive, interpersonal, and behavioral.

In actual practice, some mood-disorder patients respond well to one isolated method. For example, if the serious stress at the basis of the patient's predicament is an interpersonal problem, then efforts in psychotherapy can be directed at that problem. However, the usual approach will have mixtures of techniques. The more effective methods use combinations of behavioral, interpersonal, psychodynamic, and cognitive methods, tailored to the individual. For example, it is impossible in real life to do interpersonal psychotherapy in depth effectively without using psychodynamic concepts and principles. At present we are able to acknowledge and emphasize the usefulness of psychodynamics even though statistically it is not easy to prove.

With this summary, we are now prepared to discuss treatment of the refractory and long-term cases and demonstrate patterns that are successful.

130

PHASES OF TREATMENT

The approach of today's technique is to regard treatment as occurring in 3 phases: (1) acute, (2), continuation, and (3) maintenance (Table 6–1). Rather than plunge immediately into the long-term treatment process, first I will summarize the first 2 phases of treatment—the acute and continuation phases—to give an outline of what ought to be accomplished. Although these phases do represent what happens, they are not entirely separate. They overlap in the sense that what should be done ideally in one phase may not be accomplished until a later phase. For example, adjustment and change of medications may have to take place at any time in the treatment. Although one hopes that the most effective and satisfactory medications can be found in the acute phase, with relief of symptoms, it very often doesn't happen until later, as can be seen in the patients described later in this chapter. Another example of overlapping phases is in the use of intensive psychotherapy, which may be appropriately started early, before any medication is used. Sometimes in this situation, it is apparent after a time that medication is advisable when new symptoms appear, perhaps indicating a bipolar disorder or a major depression rather than simply a psychologically treatable problem. In that case, medication should be prescribed.

131

Table 6-1. Treatment plan and goals of treatment at each of the three treatment phases for each axis of DSM-IV-TR™

AXIS	TREATMENT PLAN	GOAL
PHASE I: ACUTE		
I. Clinical Disorders	1. Treat with medication if needed 2. Help with problems 3. Form good relationship with patient (sympathetic)	1. Relief of symptoms 2. Good, trusting relationship 3. Preliminary Multiaxial evaluation 4. Identify long-term problems, e.g., mourning
II. Personality Disorders	1. Evaluate 2. Open the door to discussion	1. Become aware of possible needs 2. Eliminate immediate problems 3. Short-term intervention
III. General Medical Conditions	1. Immediate evaluation and needed intervention 2. Consultation if needed 3. Treatment, if needed, for elimination	Eliminate the medical illness where possible as needed
IV. Psychosocial and Environmental Problems	1. Immediate intervention and help where needed 2. Eliminate problem if needed 3. Open the relationship to discussion	Eliminate trauma and stresses where needed and possible; at least to be aware and have the patient become aware that you can help and are receptive

132

V. Global Assessment of Functioning (GAF)	1. Modify and augment the treatment as needed 2. Be aware of failure of symptom relief or of failure of normal functioning	To find a combination of treatments or a treatment that brings GAF back to normal range

Preliminary Multiaxial Assessment at end of Phase I.

PHASE II: CONTINUATION

I. Clinical Disorders	1. Continue phase I treatment if successful in relief of symptoms 2. Evaluate effect of treatment and modify if needed 3. Continue open doctor-patient relationship and empathy	1. Relief of symptoms continued 2. Open the door to discussion of problems delaying recovery 3. Restore normal function if feasible 4. Assist the mourning process
II. Personality Disorders	1. Continue to evaluate any effect of personality deficit on symptoms 2. Continue to open door to empathetic relationship 3. Open door to discussion of personality problems	1. Be aware of impact and effect of any personality problems 2. Eliminate personality problems if possible at this phase

AXIS	TREATMENT PLAN	GOAL
III. General Medical Condition	1. Continue to be sure medical situation is under control 2. Treatment and consultation continued as needed	Eliminate any medical illness where needed and possible
IV. Psychosocial and Environmental Problems	1. Intervention if needed 2. Involvement of family if needed and possible 3. Work with patient when possible	Eliminate and control the effect of environmental problems and interpersonal problems
V. Global Assessment of Functioning (GAF)	1. Evaluate and be aware if functioning is not back to normal 2. If unsatisfactory, modify treatment and go on to phase III	1. Open door to patient to cooperate at looking at problems delaying recovery from symptoms 2. Observe any failure of normal function
PHASE III: MAINTENANCE		
I. Clinical Disorders	1. If some symptoms remain, go on to looking at cause in personality or environment or relationship 2. More intensive interpersonal, in-depth psychodynamic or psychoanalytic therapy 3. Change medication if needed	1. Eliminate remaining symptoms 2. Restore functioning to healthy level 3. Complete the mourning process

II. Personality Disorders	More intensive psychotherapy to look at and treat personality issues that feed into the illness	Eliminate personality pathology contributing to the chronicity and refractory illness
III. General Medical Condition	Treatment of any existing or remaining medical illness	Solve any such problems remaining
IV. Psychosocial and Environmental Problems	1. Help patient to work on any problems feeding into the illness 2. In-depth psychotherapy where needed	Solve any such problems remaining. Help patient with insight into developmental issues.
V. Global Assessment of Functioning (GAF)	1. Be aware of any remaining malfunctions 2. Treatment of causes, whether medical, personality, or psychosocial	Eliminate problems causing chronic or refractory illness as identified by the Multiaxial evaluation. (See Chapter 5.)

135

Phase I: Symptomatic Recovery

Historically, we have had to focus on the course of the acute illness. One way to understand what one can expect of the course of the various mood disorders is to look at the literature published before antidepressants became available, for example, Kraepelin's (1921) classic monograph, *Manic Depressive Insanity and Paranoia*. Here one sees that chronicity and recurrence were common in the days before more modern methods such as drugs were available to alter the natural history of the illness, but it is quite apparent from the description that we are dealing with the same illnesses as they are modified by the medications now available. It is also apparent that the illnesses can still be recurrent and chronic despite the use of effective medications that reduce symptoms and allow 50 to 65 percent of the patients to get symptomatically well. It is to that 35 to 40 percent of sufferers who do not get entirely well or stay well that this book is directed.

Phase II: Continuation and Functional Recovery

With currently available effective antidepressants, we can focus on the patients who do not recover readily symptomatically and on those whose symptoms improve but whose *functioning* is still not normal or satisfactory. After a long period of underlying illness, much of it in the developmental years, many patients have a serious need to catch up in life, both in career and in actual education and maturational development. There can be serious defects in maturation and personal life that require attention, and often it is the psychiatrist who is in a position to give them that attention, because these patients are still medicated and require attention regularly. The question often arises as to referral to a psychotherapist who can cooperate with the psychiatrist who is giving the medication and coordinating the case management. If this is done, there must still be a strong therapeutic alliance with the person managing the case.

Phase III: Maintenance

The final treatment phase involves the prolonged use of medication for prevention; continued psychotherapy, which is usually necessary; and correction of psychosocial problems with rehabilitation in cases where the long illness has prevented maturation and has limited progress toward normal goals in life.

TREATMENT AT THE THREE PHASES

Initial treatment of a depressive or manic spell depends on the symptomatic need. If medication is needed there are many antidepressants, anti-anxiety drugs, and mood levelers (see Appendix I). The latest guidelines for the treatment of patients with major depression disorder give a comprehensive description of current medications, side effects, initial and follow-up treatment (Supplement to the *American Journal of Psychiatry*, 2000, vol. 157.) That volume summarizes the current practices in enough detail to use as a reference. Psychodynamic therapy is discussed briefly but psychoanalysis is not mentioned, nor the usual practice—combined methods.

When it becomes evident that we are dealing with a chronic or treatment-resistant refractory patient, first one examines the therapeutic alliance for deficits, and then the therapeutic techniques are called into play as follows:

1. Psychopharmacological methods used for treatment-resistant, chronic, and refractory depressions.

    a. Augmentation with combinations of antidepressants.

    b. High-dose monotherapy.

    c. Changing antidepressants.

    d. Lithium augmentation.

    e. Anticonvulsants. Originally divalproex sodium (Depakote) and carbamazepine (Tegretol) were the most commonly used, but others have recently entered the therapeutic arena—Neurontin (gabapentin), Lamictal (lamotrigine).

f. Amino acids or compounds high in the amino acids involved in the serotonin metabolism. L-tryptophan, the amino-acid precursor of serotonin, had some success, but has been withdrawn from the market because of deaths; presumably due to impurities, as it had a long history of safety prior to the one batch that caused the deaths. Others in the over-the-counter market have some promise and could be useful in the future.

g. More intensive contact, with assessment, education, and increasing compliance.

h. Psychostimulants, including pergolide, bromocriptine, methylphenidate (Ritalin), and amphetamines.

2. Psychosocial treatments. Involving family, assistance in appropriate living, helping with occupational training and education.

3. Combinations and programs. Day treatment, hospitalization, team approach, family counseling, psychotherapy.

   a. Team approach. It is sometimes effective in complex situations to involve all of the influencing forces impinging on the individual. The arrangement may be similar to a method called Multi-System Therapy (Fenton 1997) that recently has evolved in the treatment of delinquent adolescents. In this approach, a well-organized team provides the treatment, with a leader doing whatever psychotherapy is needed and being available to the patient and to the other members of the team 24 hours a day, every day. The patient is never allowed to be at a loss for support, usually from one person, psychiatrist, or therapist with whom he has a bond.

b. Psychotherapeutic methods. "Can we talk?" asks a recovering patient who chastises psychiatry for too readily dismissing patients with her diagnosis (schizophrenia) as unable to benefit from talking therapy (A Recovering Patient, 1986). With managed-care administrators quick to seize upon a lack of outcome data as a pretext for limiting treatment and a public mental health system pressed to handle case loads as high as 200 to 300 patients per clinician, psychiatry's regrettable answer has often been, "No, we're too busy." And, judging by the psychiatric literature, many authoritative psychiatrists take a statistical view of therapy and ignore techniques effective in long-term therapy with characterologic disabilities. The doctor-patient relationship and the therapeutic alliance should be considered first, and then the therapy of the chronic cases we have identified has to take into account the various etiological elements that make for chronicity. So far, we have identified the following elements that contribute to chronicity:

1. Response to medication.

2. Personality deficits.

    a. Deficit in judgment

    b. Interpersonal problems, failures of identification

    c. Pathological ideas

3. Early losses or traumas.

4. Functioning deficits.

5. Comorbidity.

6. Current losses or traumas.

4. Rehabilitation. During the years of chronicity the patient may have lost so much in career, personal life, productivity, and goals in life, that he or she needs to make progress in catching up. The techniques involved in this will be illustrated in the case examples: the first

case a woman with bipolar II, finding the ultimate successful career in marriage and motherhood; the second case an early-middle-aged man returning to school to find an appropriate career and to improve his status as a provider for his family; and the third case a patient who was able to go back to school and with rehabilitation find a successful and happy career. The physician's function and the therapeutic alliance will be illustrated in the case examples.

To see how these treatment techniques can be used in combination, we will examine long-term, chronic cases in the next chapter.

To illustrate some of the techniques needed in the rehabilitation process, see the two letters in Appendix II. They involve "going to bat" for the patient with his insurance source. You won't get everything you want and recommend, but you may get enough to get the patient's treatment established in the present. The future may require more. Most of the letters I have written have secured some additional time for therapy, but it is a far cry from the earlier days, when the needs of the patient dictated the type, length, and intensity of therapy.

7

Case Examples of the Treatment of Chronic Mood Disorders

INTRODUCTION TO THE CASE EXAMPLES

This book has been aimed at the long-standing problem of chronicity and refractoriness in mood disorders. A rather complex method of identifying the clinical factors responsible for this problem, using the Multiaxial System (DSM-IV-TR™ 2000, p. 27 ff.) of scoring the severity and identifying etiological factors, has been presented. Some practitioners will find it unnecessary to use such a complex method, but it will at least direct the clinician's attention to the issues feeding into any particular patient's chronicity and can open the door to solving the problem. The method of treatment will depend on what is uncovered in working with the patient. The importance of the issues comprising the predicament—the problems facing the patient and leading him or her into a mood disorder or illness—will become apparent and will affect the treatment methods chosen.

The case reports that follow illustrate the usefulness and the necessity of long-term treatment of sufficient intensity to eradicate and override long-standing symptoms. They illustrate the effectiveness and complexity of combined methods—medication; psychotherapy of a complex nature; psychosocial intervention; plus the formation of an effective patient-physician relationship, which becomes an alliance. The case reports further illustrate that limiting the psychotherapeutic sessions in number and frequency will result in failure to cure, thus increasing the overall cost and prolonging the treatment process.

The combined methods of psychotherapy include psychoanalytic, cognitive, interpersonal, behavioral, and relationship techniques—whatever is appropriate to the situation. "Combined" means together with medication but also means combinations of techniques. For example, a therapist may give guidance and advice to a patient and also analyze the origin of a symptom in early life as in psychoanalysis, at the same time requiring analysis of the transference relationship with the patient. The patients in my chronic series who have done best in the long run are those who had a standard psychoanalysis in addition to whatever else was required. The cases also illustrate the present-day awareness that psychotherapy can overcome long-standing, seemingly ingrained, character traits and symptoms left untouched by drug treatment. Further, psychotherapy frees up the patient from those symptoms and allows whatever rehabilitation and catching up is desirable.

REFERENCES TO THE BASIC MODEL OF THERAPY IN THE BOOK

In this book, we have been dealing with the modern, currently standard, symptomatically diagnosed mood disorders. The descriptive diagnostic approach has been the basis of identifying and treating patients classified as having mood disorders (Frank and Kupfer 2000). "Use of Clinical Judgment" (*Diagnostic and Statistical Manual*, DSM-IV-TR, p. xxxii). "It is important that DSM-IV not be applied mechanically by untrained individuals. The specific diagnostic criteria included in the manual are meant to serve as guidelines to be enforced by clinical judgment and are not meant to be used in cookbook fashion" (*Diagnostic and Statistical Manual* 2000, p. xxxii).

The developmental approach of the predicament as defined in Chapter 5 has been the basis of my description of the current clinical treatment intervention I used. The January 2000 *Archives of General*

Psychiatry had 3 articles on prospects for the twenty-first century, based on what has been learned recently about the body-mind interaction. These articles shed light on why the current methods described in this book can work to eliminate even the long-standing, chronic, seemingly refractory mood disorders. In one of those articles, Kupfer and Frank (2000) ask, "How does life experience alter gene expression in vulnerable individuals?" and "What are the neurobiological effects of psychotherapy?" Akil and Watson (2000, p. 88) state that, "The tension between the biomedical and the psychotherapeutic approaches in psychiatry needs to be eliminated and transformed in a fully integrated approach that is mindful of the biological, emotional, cognitive, and social complexity of each individual." They further state (Akil and Watson 2000, p. 87), "We need to comprehend how experience in the human brain including social interactions modify particular circuits in reversible and irreversible ways" and that "Social interactions, and therefore talking therapies, can change brain structure and function just as drugs do." In the same issue, Hyman (2000, pp. 88–89) wrote, "Everything we learn—a process dependent both on particular circuits and on regulation of particular genes—physically changes the brain." The origin of personality attributes is described by Shore (1994) in his book *Affect Regulation and the Origin of Self: Neurology of Emotional Development.*

THE BASIC MODEL—
MEDICATION PLUS PSYCHOTHERAPY

A neurophysiologist can see the fixed behavior, such as symptoms of depression, as based on an abnormality of fixed circuitry in the brain, of course using neurochemical substrates. To alter these circuits and replace them with more normal circuitry requires overriding the pathological circuitry with more normal circuitry and patterns of behavior, mood, and thinking. In a well-established pathological disorder, this is made possible by using medication to loosen hold of the fixed pathological circuitry on behavior patterns. For example, I have found that using either clomipramine (Anafranil) or fluvoxamine maleate (Luvox) for obsessive-compulsive disorder (OCD) to loosen the hold that a pathological circuit has on behavior and then substituting normal behavior little by little will produce a more normal circuitry. It can take time— e.g., 2 years or more—to do this, plus intensive psychotherapeutic work focusing on behavior.

The same model is at the basis of the changes induced in the cases of mood disorders described in this book: medication was used to loosen the hold that chronic, habitual circuitry has; then a more normal circuitry was established over time, a period that may take years using psychotherapeutic methods.

147

The Uncovering of Causes
of the Abnormal Circuitry

Often the chronic pathological mood is relieved by these procedures, and then the patient has an increased awareness of what experiences in his life may have influenced the course of the mood. For example, one depressed patient who had developed a panic when exposed to crowds, upon being able with treatment to tolerate crowds, remembered one incident in childhood, his first panic attack, when he was locked out of the house nude accidentally for several hours and became panicky.

In conclusion, it needs to be said that most of the refractory and chronic mood disorders can be helped and relieved of symptoms by intensive and thorough technical treatment, using the basic model of medication plus psychotherapy.

CASE EXAMPLES

Nowadays one sometimes finds a case that illustrates in dramatic detail the re-enactment of early losses and traumas. Before antidepressants, it could often be seen very realistically and dramatically in patients in psychoanalysis. Therefore, to start, I present an analyzed case from the days before we had specific antidepressants. This is a case I can present in some detail without the danger of violation of privacy because the patient is long deceased as a result of an intercurrent, unrelated, medical problem. In addition to illustrating the importance of childhood losses and traumas, this case also demonstrates some of the personality problems that are an essential part of the predicament and how they can be worked through and relieved in an intensive psychodynamic treatment like psychoanalysis. I considered those symptoms that were relieved by medication as symptoms of the depression and not of deeply ingrained personality problems. The other part of the predicament—i.e., the need for someone to supply the comfort, love, security, attachment—eventually was solved when a loving, kind husband with many parental protective qualities met that need and completed the solving of the predicament.

First Chronic Patient (Patient A)

In 1946, the young woman came to our low-fee clinic with the aftermath of a depression severe enough to disable her from her work in the Women's Army Corps as a skilled nurse's aide. I took her into once-a-week therapy, which did not solve her downhill course. She had to be admitted to the hospital, where she was given eight electroconvulsant treatments, bringing about complete remission. Because of the history of previous depression and because she had personal issues involving her family and her husband of a few months, I then took her into standard psychoanalysis on a basis

149

of 5 days a week. She was one of the people who can talk volubly throughout a depression, and this made it possible for the "working through" of her early traumas, griefs, identifications, and subsequent personality problems.

The following is a summary of the main experiences she "worked through" over a period of 5 years. In the first 4 years, she had to be admitted to the hospital 3 times for electroconvulsant therapy, which brought her out of the depression but into a state of hyperexcitement, which turned out to be hypomanic, with poor judgment and overstimulation sexually. We now call it Bipolar II. Although the cyclical symptoms were controlled and she was no longer manic or depressed, it became apparent that she was still disabled and not functioning in a normal, healthy, realistic way. What remained seemed to be personality traits of long standing, which surfaced and dominated her behavior once the illness was controlled. These traits included a tendency to be dominated in her behavior by wishful fantasies, hypersensitivity to others, overwhelmingly low self-esteem, passivity, and submissiveness alternating with rebellion. What was needed was a way to bring her to a more normal, healthier-functioning state.

Nowadays, with patients this severely ill, we try to relieve the symptoms but also hope to cover up or override the psychology with medication, especially the anticonvulsants, which usually can control the mania or hypomania but do not always correct the poor judgment and childhood fixations that can cause a lot of troubles. Today, she would be prescribed one or more of these: valproic acid (Depakote), carbamazepine (Tegretol), lamotrigine (Lamictal), lithium, verapamil (Calan, etc.), temazepam (Restoril), gabapentine (Neurontin). At that time, before these medications were available to alter the picture, it was possible to see what working through in psychoanalytic therapy, with no time limit, would do. We had the help of the family: the mother had died when the patient was 12 but the father and sister took care of her when she was unable, so she had a caring family environment, although the absence of a loving mother was a powerful part of the predicament.

The following are the principal character problems caused by early losses—traumas "worked through" in the analysis. The transference was not analyzed as thoroughly as it would be nowadays, but transference issues came to the surface and were re-experienced dramatically.

1. *Emotions (rage).* Her anger and aggression against men, particularly her father, came out first, then was turned on me as she developed a transference relationship as I became the most important man in her life, as her father had been. Thus, it became possible to work it through as part of the present, and not just a remote and obscure memory of childhood. Many sessions consisted of my simply listening to the flood of anger over her childhood

151

deprivations, real and fantasized. The turning of the tide came when I increased her hours from 2 to 5 a week. Then, although gratified, her anger became more specific. The reason she was angry was that as a father figure, I allowed her to get into an affair with a man and get hurt. For the first time, it seemed possible to bring her out of chaos as she showed signs of developing a positive transference, giving us a chance to mobilize her childhood relationship with her parents, including mourning for her mother that had been hidden by her sexual overstimulation.

2. *Anxiety*. In the hospital, she became aware of homosexual feelings toward the woman who was her roommate, wanting to touch her body. This created such anxiety about being close to the woman and such curiosity about the woman's body that she decided that she would be more comfortable outside the hospital. It awakened memories of her mother's body in the bathtub and the large breasts, and memories of sleeping close to her sister in the same bed. She tried to read neutral literature, which would take her away from sexuality and dirt.

3. *Defenses*. She developed a hand-washing compulsion in the hospital. In her analytic work

this became associated with her father's hand on her mother's body—a very "dirty" thing to do. One of the things that emerged in the analysis was the vividness of her visual fantasies—not hallucinatory but sometimes operating as something she could cling to, to keep her from being alone with her feelings.

4. *Sexuality*. Very active sexual excitement fantasies emerged when she left the hospital, apparently in a somewhat hypomanic state. However, it turned out that she was not only anorgasmic but entirely frigid, and the fantasies were of crawling up on the analyst's lap and searching his pockets. Apparently, her sexual fantasies were still at an almost infantile level. Her choice was for passive men, as she was so readily aroused sexually.

5. A *sense of helplessness* was found to be an undercurrent motivating her to become very passive in the early stages of the depression.

6. *Positive feelings* began to grow in the transference, and she had the fantasy of paying the analyst with the only coin she had, which was herself.

7. *Defenses*. After 2½ years of analysis, she continued to have periods of depression through which the analysis was now able to continue,

and her defenses could be analyzed. These were chiefly: 1) projections, 2) acting out, and 3) regression. For example, she accused most men of mother fixations, a very strong characteristic of herself, and a basic force in the predicament, i.e., the need in childhood for the loving and protective mother. Because her mother had chronic heart disease throughout the patient's childhood, she could not supply this. An example of regression came after an injection of penicillin in her buttocks. Her associations were seeing her mother nude in the bathtub and being attracted to her mother's large breasts. She related this to her fantasies of fellatio, which fantasies had troubled her in going out with men. An example of acting out her fantasies came when she was dating a man. She spoke of him as her "fiancé," until she discovered that he had no intension of marrying her. After two more years of analysis, she began to be "petrified" with fear of coming to the analysis, for fear of attacking the analyst. She felt "like a dog in heat." Fantasies of fellatio during the analytic session were so strong she had to sit up to get away from the ideas.

8. *Work.* When she left the hospital to go back to work, she said, "Work is not important, what is important is to be looked after."

9. *Termination.* After another year of concentrated analysis, the spells of depression became milder and did not again require electroconvulsant therapy. She had two mild spells, one related to her husband's resistance to her desire to have a child. She worked through this with him when he became aware that she probably could do this without endangering her health. The second depression came when her sister became ill and this allowed her to work through some feelings about the sister. It appears that the new self—motherhood, being a house-wife, writing poetry—was a happier self than the ambitious, competitive self she was before entering analysis. Shortly afterward she moved out of town and was outside of my care, but occasionally in a Christmas card would report that she was happy, was staying at home, was raising her child, and the marriage was happy. The husband was a loving, protective parent both to their son and to her. The predicament was relieved.

10. *Follow-up.* Thirty-five years later, I wrote her as one of a group on whom I was doing a follow-up, and she sent a letter from a distant city with the statement, "I still take medicine, but as far as I am concerned, my analysis saved my life. I would either be dead or in the hospital without the analysis."

The early sexual attachment covered up much of any open mourning for the absence of mothering due to her mother's long illness and ultimate death when the patient was about to enter adolescence. However, after working through these attachments in the transference, she was able to develop a strong mother identification and conquer her hidden grief by becoming a mother herself.

Working through is the process not only of recovering the memory but reliving the emotions attached to the memory. In psychoanalysis, this process occurs in connection with the transference: i.e., the process whereby what was felt early in life is transferred to the analyst within the analytic hour, verbalized, felt, re-experienced, and then eliminated as a symptom. It is possible that an abbreviated form of therapy, such as the type of therapy described by McCullough (see Chapter 6), might do much the same thing, although the "working through" in the conventional analysis seems much more thorough and may result in a longer persistence of therapeutic results.

The use of medicines has made working through possible in patients who before medication could not complete the process. This patient represents a group able to work through her illness when the symptoms were controlled with electroconvulsant therapy. Nowadays, modern drugs are able to control the symptoms sufficiently to use psychotherapy for the underlying psychological problems.

The Multiaxial system was not yet formulated when this patient was treated, but in retrospect, it is worthwhile to do an assessment of her from the history, as it reveals the basic clinical reasons why her ultimately successful treatment was arranged, and why it turned out successfully. The assessment at the time, expressed in up-to-date terms, i.e., a Multiaxial assessment, follows:

Patient A	
Score	**Treatment Plan**
Negative Factors	
AXIS I. Score 10. Diagnosis: Bipolar I and II. At times disabling depressions, alternating with elevated mood to the extent that her judgment was bad and she was sexually overactive. Probably more bipolar II than I.	Hospitalization with electroconvulsant treatments when serious depression occurred. Family intervention when needed. Medication.
AXIS II. Score 10. Personality disorder, mixed, with dependent, paranoid, and other features of failure to mature, in addition to the poor judgment of the hypomanic state she sometimes showed when recovering from a depression.	Psychoanalysis, 5 days a week.
AXIS III. Score 0. No medical problems.	Not needed.

AXIS IV. Score 5. Psychosocial and environmental problems. Family conflicts. Not much attention or supervision by father. Mother died when the patient was 12. Not satisfied with career. Divorced from husband; no "important other."	1. Family intervention when needed. Intensive "working through," in analysis, of the early losses and traumas.
AXIS V. Score 10. Global assessment of functioning unpredictable. Goes from 40 to 50 depending on phase of illness. Never higher, even when out of depression or hypomanic state.	Continue psychoanalysis as needed.

TOTAL NEGATIVE FACTORS: 35 (Predicament Present)

POSITIVE FACTORS

Cooperative with treatment: Score 10.	Able to form good doctor-patient relationship.
Family support good: Score 10.	Family helpful when needed. She had a home and was looked after when unable to support herself. Remarried happily.
Response to treatment: Score 5.	Good response to electroconvulsant treatment; complete recovery from depressions.
Ability to carry out treatment: Score 10.	Treatment could be as intensive as needed. Could complete analysis.

TOTAL POSITIVE FACTORS: 35
NET SCORE (NEGATIVE minus POSITIVE): 0
Predicament solved through analysis plus finding a husband and protector.
COMMENTS: It is evident in retrospect that it appeared worthwhile to the psychiatrist at the time that intensive therapy was needed to back up the electroconvulsant treatment that brought her out of her disabling depressions. At the time, psychoanalysis was used intensively for her personality problems, and she was fortunate enough to be able to have this treatment. In addition, the new medications control her inherited bipolar symptoms, allowing the analytic results to continue positively, and keep her predicament solved.

MEDICATION USE IN PSYCHOANALYSIS

It is becoming more evident that in a standard psychoanalysis, symptoms may arise that create blocks to the progress of the analysis that can be removed by use of standard medication, and the analysis can continue successfully. The psychoanalytic literature contains some examples. I will summarize 2 of these examples; the first example is of a report of 7 cases of bipolar illness under good control (Loeb and Loeb 1987).

The 7 patients in analysis were being treated with lithium. The authors observed that psychoanalysis and analytic psychotherapy enabled the patients to become aware of their previously unconscious phallic wishes and impulses and how increased doses of lithium at that point permitted them to avoid manic attacks by counteracting those inappropriate sexual inclinations. Lithium made possible this awareness of the increased sexual drive before it could be acted out. The lithium level was found to have dropped at this point, indicating the beginning of a manic attack. When this was discovered, the dose of lithium was increased, raising the blood level to the therapeutic level, and the sexual drive lessened to a normal intensity. Thus, inappropriate behavior was avoided during the analysis by the use of lithium. This remarkable technique increases the availability of analysis for bipolar patients who might need it.

But what about the cases we are used to having in analysis, those without a major disorder—the nonpsychotic, functioning, everyday patient who is not happy with himself and is not functioning up to his capacity and talents; who is either overinhibited, escapist, or mildly depressed; who is unable to form satisfactory relationships and wonders why, etc. He is or has been in treatment, but is lonely and wonders what is wrong with these relationships and is seriously enough discontented to be very concerned about what might be wrong with him. Here now is such a case, summarized from Wylie and Wylie (1987).

The patient was a 39-year old divorced woman with 2 apparently normal adolescent children and a good job as an administrator, a job she was beginning to find "lackadaisical." In the 7 years since her divorce, she had not been able to establish a satisfactory long-term relationship with a man. This appeared remarkable, because she was attractive, socially engaging, educated, and had many friends. She complained of intermittent periods of depression also. She appeared very suitable for psychoanalysis. In the initial interview, it appeared that she had struggled for years with intermittent, noncyclical episodes of depressed mood. Various of her physicians had prescribed amphetamines for fatigue and mood disturbances. Before the *Diagnostic and Statistical Manuals*, this would have been a depressive neurosis. Nowadays, it is dysthymia.

A trial of tricyclics had not been effective, nor had a brief period of psychotherapy. In finding her suitable for analysis, the analyst saw that she had been a successful mother; had enabled the children to have a good relationship with the father; and had a capacity for self-reflection, a capacity for sublimation, and evidence for interpersonal constancy, even though she seemed to choose inappropriate men. Other forms of therapy had only been temporarily successful.

The first year went very well, and she entered the analytic process readily. However, analysis of transference met persistent obstacles, such as her response to a transference interpretation, that she could not "imagine such things." Throughout the next year, it became evident that there was a serious obstacle to forming a therapeutic relationship that could be analyzed, and, at the same time, she was struggling with recurrent feelings of depression. The analyst observed that his pattern was similar to her history of an "atypical" depression—recurrent attacks of depressed mood when rejected, eating or using alcohol to relieve the feeling, a lack of response to tricyclics, etc.

The standard drug type used for atypical depression is the MAO inhibitor class; it was decided that analysis alone would not work well, and phenelzine, a drug of that class, was started.

She remained on the drug for 10 months, during which time all other aspects of the analysis remained unchanged. However, in contrast, within a month, it became possible for her to acknowledge her feelings for the analyst, finding him as attractive as the suitable men "with whom she had been afraid to seek a relationship." She soon was able to describe how she had found a need in the past "to stumble through various past relationships." She was able often to describe her feelings in this connection, a very important issue. Analysis of transference feelings were thereafter analyzed whenever they became appropriate. In addition, her dependency on food decreased, she was more assertive in her work, and she began to enjoy things that had previously bored her.

During the year that followed, it was possible to work through memories, recollections, and feelings that surfaced, such as frightening thoughts and fantasies that had lain behind her difficulty in functioning in her personal relationships. About a year after the end of the drug trial, she was able to form a solid relationship with a suitable man and was enjoying it.

In summary, Wylie and Wylie (1987) felt that the drug made it possible to analyze material essential to work through the patient's problems, material that otherwise would have been inaccessible. This is an example of a patient formerly unable to complete an analysis, for whom analysis is now available.

Rehabilitation

Second Chronic Patient (Today's Patient) (Patient B)

I have chosen to describe this patient as she represents the course and treatment of a bipolar schizoaffective patient who had the benefit of modern treatment techniques, plus the ability to use the doctor-patient relationship in a constructive way, allowing working through of long-standing personality problems in a psychodynamic, supportive therapy. Rehabilitation then became possible.

The case illustrates a typical chronic and recurrent schizoaffective disorder with episodic psychosis in a young, gifted adult, starting in adolescence; treated with combined therapy with both individual and team therapy and polypharmacy and ending with a rehabilitation program designed to bring the patient back into the mainstream of society. The individual therapy was fairly intensive, combining supportive, directive, interpersonal, and psychodynamic therapy applied in a manner based on the patient's condition at any given time and on the phase of the illness: a technique very much like that described by Fenton (1997) for schizophrenics, with the therapy varying according to the type and phase of the illness. The system described by McCullough (2000) resembles this treatment.

This is a woman of educated family, now 38 years old, whose illness started when she was 16 years old and continued off and on with several hospital admissions for episodes of major psychotic depression treated vigorously with standard medications, including large doses of Selective Serotonin Reuptake Inhibitors (SSRIs), despite which standard treatment she continued to require periodic hospitalization until 6 years ago at age 32, when she was started on the antipsychotic drug clozapine. After about a year of gradually increasing the dose, an adequate blood level of clozapine of about 500–600+ mg/ml had been reached, there were no breakdowns or hospital admissions for the next 5 years. During these years, she has been seen weekly in the clinic where the clozapine was given. Also, the psychiatrist who monitored the program was available at all times, did psychotherapy at least one hour a week, and dealt with all personal issues and problems complicating her rehabilitation back to the mainstream of society. After all this, she is a woman who has had numerous severe depressive episodes over a period of 15 years, from adolescence until age 32 and between times had not functioned well, had only worked sporadically at low-level jobs, had not finished school, and had no specialized training for a career. She had not learned to function well in society or in interpersonal relations; in fact had never had any long-standing personal relationships, and had never had a serious male relationship.

Prepsychotic Phase: Her adolescence was complicated by marijuana and other drugs. There was one bright spot in those years—namely, when she was first hospitalized at age 16, she was considered schizophrenic but had a psychoanalytically oriented psychiatrist who specialized in treatment of adolescents. He treated her psychotherapeutically with a fairly intensive psychotherapy, supportive but with strong psychodynamic elements, over a period of 6 or 7 years, giving her insights into herself that later turned out to be of great help once her illness was under control. Also, family support was excellent throughout her illness.

First Psychotic Phase: When her *first adult psychotic break* occurred at age 26, she was wandering through the South and was hospitalized once there. Upon release she came home and sought the child psychoanalyst who had seen her through her adolescence. He referred her to a psychoanalytically trained psychiatrist who immediately took her into treatment, and a standard intensive program was started, using antidepressants and biweekly office sessions. It was apparent that her breakdown had been a depression with psychotic elements: a schizoaffective psychosis, bipolar type.

She now has to "grow up," since her psychosis is now under control with clozapine, and her earlier psychodynamic and behavioral psychotherapy has turned out to be very helpful. She is now back in college at the point where she dropped out 20 years earlier, attending about two-thirds of a full-time schedule but successful in the work she is able to do. She is able to live by herself, fraternize with people, and participate in a rehabilitation program requiring attendance at weekly group sessions. She is very reliable in attendance in her individual weekly therapy sessions and often calls between them for advice about some personal issue. It became apparent that there was a lack of confidence in her own decisions about people, about courses to take, about the essays she writes to complete an assignment, though she is an excellent writer and has a remarkable grasp of the material. Concentration is still a problem in the sense that she seems unable to take a full schedule and has considerable anxiety from day to day about the work. Despite this anxiety, she has begun to take charge of her own life and has been able to overcome some of the inferiority she grew up with and has developed a capacity to make firm decisions of her own. This is quite a change from the submissiveness of earlier years. It is as if she is at last grown up.

PHASE I. *Treatment of Symptoms: Prepsychotic period, age 16 to about 30.*

Diagnosis: During the first psychiatric hospital admission at age 16, although not grossly psychotic, she was showing signs of becoming alienated from her family, who were highly educated and successful. The diagnosis of the psychologist was paranoid schizophrenia, based on his examination and the results of the

Minnesota Multiphasic Personality Inventory, the Rorschach Test, and the Thematic Apperception Test. A marked paranoid flavor dominated her thinking. She showed altered concentration and attention.

Although not so apparent clinically, her reality testing was seriously impaired. Her attitudes were more likely to be based on fantasy rather than reality. As an adolescent, she was diagnosed as psychotic. She was treated with trifluoperazine (Stelazine) and was for the next 7 years treated by the psychoanalyst who specialized in treatment of adolescents.

First Treatment, age 16 to 23. The psychotherapy was of a mixed type, with behavioral, counseling and psychodynamic techniques. Under this therapy the patient was able, for the first time, to give up marijuana and to take a job. She then worked at various simple service jobs—waitress, clerical, checkout clerk at a grocery store. Because of her odd appearance with disheveled hair and street clothing she was teased a great deal, often got angry, and never held a job more than a few weeks or months, usually getting fired. She was able to get another job because she was well-spoken, seemed polite and intelligent despite her appearance, which actually was not unusual during the "hippie" era of that time, even in young people who came from educated, professional families. Years later she was able to use the insights she gained in this treatment to understand and control her behavior once her psychosis was under control with medication.

PHASE 1. Psychotic period:

Treatment: hospitalization with rapid reduction of symptoms with medication, followed by psychosocial intervention (involvement of family, use of community facilities, establishing a therapeutic alliance, supportive psychotherapy, cognitive and interpersonal therapy where appropriate).

First psychotic episode. At age 26, with some money she had saved, she bussed and bummed her way to Florida with a group. When she got there, she tried to work, but was too sick to hold a job. She was admitted to a hospital on the basis of some delusions, such as that she was surrounded by a force field, and that she felt that she was on LSD, which she was not. She felt that the hospital staff were torturing her and felt overwhelmed by panic. When released after 10 days, she still had severe anxiety, to the point of panic. She came home to live with her parents. At that time she still looked unkempt, was very depressed, had ideas of reference, could not concentrate although intellectually intact, and easily became panicky when around people. She avoided public toilets, high buildings, and closed places. At that time she fit into the diagnosis of schizoaffective psychosis, atypical, with a personality that could be considered borderline. In addition, she had a clear-cut anxiety disorder with phobias.

She was able to form a relationship with the psychiatrist who saw her at least once a week, and between times received and answered numerous phone calls from the patient, asking for reassurance and guidance. She was given amitriptyline and propanolol; and, because she began to have upswings of mood with erotomania, and irritability to the point of belligerence, the medication was changed to 1200 mg of lithium, 12 mg of perphenazine, 150 mg of doxepin, and 1 mg of lorazepam. She was now 31 years old and was clearly suffering from a chronic cycling bipolar illness with additional schizoid-psychotic symptoms and a chronic anxiety disorder with phobias and obsessive symptoms. However, she was intellectually intact, was able to take college courses, and was able to work in a psychotherapeutic relationship with her psychiatrist. It turned out that she was a gifted musician and was able to enroll in music school and study her instrument seriously although with many misgivings on her part, requiring a great deal of support and encouragement from the therapist as a factor in the rehabilitation.

The predicament was temporarily solved by having a male therapist who substituted for the "significant other," giving her the care she needed for support and temporarily holding off the anxiety caused by the lack of a mother figure. However, she has now requested a woman therapist because she has some problems she needs to work through with a mother substitute, thus solving the predicament and eliminating the underlying cause. The Multiaxial evaluation shows a good prognosis despite a high score of negative factors. These were balanced against a high score in positive factors, indicating a good prognosis.

Patient B	
DSM-IV Multiaxial evaluation applied retroactively	
Score	**Treatment Plan**
Negative Factors	
AXIS I. Score 10. Diagnosis: Schizoaffective disorder, depressed with some psychotic symptoms (history) anxiety disorder with phobias. History of marijuana use in adolescence.	1. Form good doctor-patient relationship. Use medication to control depression and phobia. Enlist cooperation of family. Refer to mood clinic for clozepine when needed.
AXIS II. Score 5. Personality disorder: Some dependency and paranoid features, but reliable and dedicated to treatment.	1. Supervise behavior through counseling. Insight therapy when symptoms are controlled. Use the psychoanalytic insights from previous therapy.
AXIS III. Score 0. No medical problems.	
AXIS IV. Score 8. Environmental and psychosocial problems. Dropped out of school in adolescence. No job or special skills.	1. Assist in rehabilitation through social agency. Return to school when able.
AXIS V. Score 8. Global Assessment of Functioning: unable to work but can come to therapy. Cooperative.	

TOTAL NEGATIVE FACTORS: 33	
Serious predicament at the start of treatment.	
POSITIVE FACTORS	
(Including those that developed later to solve the predicament)	
Early psychotherapy: Score 5.	Good response to therapy in adolescence with some insight retained.
Strong depressive element in symptoms: Score 5.	Very cooperative in treatment—able to form a strong treatment alliance.
Lack of psychotic symptoms at present: Score 5.	Free of psychosis with medication (clozapine).
Family history: Score 5.	
Family support: Score 5.	Very helpful.
Cooperative Family: Score 5.	Very helpful.
TOTAL POSITIVE FACTORS: 30	
NET SCORE (NEGATIVE minus POSITIVE): 3	
PREDICAMENT: No predicament at present.	

PHASE 2. Post-Psychotic Period.

This phase involved treatment of the patient's functioning in society. Psychotherapy was continued as during the acute psychosis. The depressive symptoms were much fewer, and she was compliant with all treatment modalities. The patient also attended daily sessions in partial hospitalization. She had increasing insights into the psychology of her illness. The therapy included some work on childhood development and psychodynamic insights. This period lasted several months.

During this period she was very compliant with medication, able to socialize with persons in the group, and able to live at home with her father and mother; but it became apparent that she had impulses to harm herself, was very sensitive to slights, and took offense easily. She got rid of some of the impulses and pathological fantasies by drawing and painting impressionistic and abstract works and by playing tremendously emotional music on her instrument, getting a good deal of satisfaction and some relief of anxiety by externalizing and thus sublimating her anger.

PHASE 3. CHRONIC PHASE.
Growth and maturation.

Subsequent Course. Over the next 5 years she continued to be under intensive treatment, with weekly and twice-weekly therapeutic sessions with her psychiatrist, and with intensive treatment of her phobias. She was participating in group therapy and attended a self-help group weekly, but despite medication had to be treated more intensively six times for suicidal thoughts severe enough to cause panic, or for impulses to cut or otherwise harm herself, as for example the impulse to cut her wrists. Each time she was able to get under control within a few days, when admitted to the hospital. The hospital atmosphere apparently gave her comfort in a variety of ways and did not arouse the sadistic impulses and self-destructive feelings that burgeoned in the outside world. There was no change in the medication in the hospital, but family visits in that atmosphere were very comforting. Comfort and love supplied the missing security needed.

Medication. During those 5 years she tended to develop extrapyramidal symptoms severe enough to require a change of the antipsychotic medication. Thiothixene, trifluoperazine, and perphenazine all caused sufficiently severe symptoms to require a change, and did not control the prepsychotic behavior that repeatedly landed her in the hospital.

At this point a critical decision was made—to treat her with the atypical antipsychotic drug clozapine (Clozaril), because her psychotic episodes kept recurring. This gave added structure to her life because of the need for frequent blood counts and weekly examination. Lithium was discontinued and Depakote (divalproex sodium) started, along with sertraline (Zoloft) in doses up to 400 mg daily. Because of her severe anxiety symptoms clonazepam (Klonopin) was prescribed, with considerable relief. The sadistic and self-destructive impulses have been reduced to a manageable degree, but other comorbid symptoms have become more evident. In the several years since clozapine was started, she has not had to be admitted to the hospital and has been able to go back to school and take courses that will lead to a degree in accounting.

Psychotherapy. However, with the cycling under control, two problems have surfaced—her phobias and anxieties, and character and interpersonal problems that cause considerable trouble and prevent her from getting solid rehabilitation. For these symptoms, the psychotherapeutic sessions have continued consistently, at least once a week, but are now based on insight rather than counseling. For example, she was troubled because she thought her stringed instrument was out of tune and she was going to get someone else to tune it; but she remembered that during her therapy as an adolescent, her therapist, a psychoanalyst, pointed out that she had always depended too much on her mother. With that in mind she decided to tune it herself, which she did, quite successfully.

PHASE 3. Maturation. Overcoming long-standing character traits. Chronic Phase continues. Rehabilitation.

(Returning to the social mainstream, functioning normally, having more normal interpersonal relations. In brief, achieving a *functional recovery*.)

The question arises when the symptoms of the illness are brought under control with medication, "can this person be rehabilitated and restored to normal—meaning, brought back into the mainstream of society, live a normal life"? This is especially important in the severely ill, like this patient, where her long-term illness has prevented her from getting an education of the kind that would enable her to become self-supporting; and has prevented her from maturing in character, attitudes, and personal relationships. She was overly sensitive; not exactly paranoid, but easily offended. The question also arises as to whether the illness is of a deteriorating type. When she had reached the point where she could concentrate on tasks such as learning a complicated piece of music or reading a book, at that point she was referred to the Bureau of Rehabilitation, through which she was able to enroll in an excellent music school, starting on a part-time basis.

Another therapeutic move was made at her own suggestion. She asked to see a female therapist and had weekly sessions with her, which brought out some of the developmental experiences she had failed to make with her mother. The memory of the relationship with her mother brought out some insight into changes she needed to make in herself—for example, the need to be more assertive and to take firmer control of her own life, rather than being so passive and submissive. It was as if her role as a dependent had continued into adult life, and she was now ready to take charge of her own life. A new self emerged—an adult self. She no longer had to treat the infantile self she had been with marijuana. She had "grown up," and the personality problems that were a part of the predicament had been solved.

The basis of therapy through all phases of treatment has been to treat the patient as a person, with empathy. *Phase 1: Relief of Symptoms.* Medication (including clozapine) and close supervision by the mood clinic, with additional weekly hour-long sessions with the individual psychiatrist of management, family contact when needed, and hospitalization when needed. Functioning still at a dependent level—outside of the mainstream of society. *Phase 2: Functioning in Society.* This phase started when she went on clozapine. Phasing back into society with courses at college. Continuation of medication and contact with the hospital clozapine clinic, plus intensive psychotherapy with one or two weekly hour-long sessions with her personal psychiatrist. This required her to plan, pay close attention to her functioning level, and be able to internalize the respect she was shown. She has used the therapist as a source of approval for growth and maturation. The therapy is a mixture of interpersonal, cognitive, and psychodynamic, but with reality counseling always at the basis, because of her tendency to be unrealistic and overly sensitive. *Improvement in judgment.* This phase overlapped with the next phase. *Phase 3: Maturation.* Attention to the self, overcoming long-standing personality problems—shyness, sensitivity, fears, dependency, with weekly hour-long sessions of psychodynamic and interpersonal therapy. Reality counseling was not as necessary because of the improvement in her judgment. Adding a female therapist for identification purposes, with weekly sessions, resulted in her being able to take charge of her own life and to change her role from that of a dependent to an independent person. The time required for this change has been 5 years since her psychotic spells have been eliminated with clozapine.

However, the process of rehabilitation would still have had to follow its course, with treatment of her phobias, with counseling, with the acquiring of insight into her problems in interpersonal relations, with her acquiring self-respect and a better grasp of realistic thinking, and finally, the maturation from dependency to taking charge of her own life. The clozapine response made this possible by controlling the cycling and the psychotic tendency.

In addition, this progress would not have been possible without the various facilities available—a clozapine clinic, a day-treatment clinic, a state-funded rehabilitation agency, a family that could be relied on to help with practical matters such as getting a car for transportation, a government that gives support to the disabled, a dedicated, psychoanalytically trained psychiatrist who coordinated the whole process, and a patient with the potential to develop.

This is an example of an originally chronic and refractory patient who was intensively treated and closely followed. It shows the kind of investment that has to be made to bring some of the sicker and more disabled patients with a psychotic disorder back into the mainstream. An effective treatment with medication to relieve the psychotic symptoms made the subsequent psychotherapeutic development possible. We do not know whether she will become entirely well eventually, although she passes for well out in the world now. It is possible that she will become self-supporting. The predicament is eliminated as an underlying cause.

The diagnosis of her psychosis in the current terminology (American Psychiatric Association 2000) is schizoaffective psychosis. She also was phobic and had a dependent personality. However, the capacity to be dedicated and consistent in the therapy showed a personality strength that allowed her to use therapy to solve the problems by constancy in the therapy, by reliability, and by the formation of a therapeutic alliance. The strong need for a mother figure is not entirely eliminated, but work on this issue is continuing. There were some of the elements of the manic state in which she became speeded-up and grandiose, had insomnia, and became somewhat overstimulated sexually; but at the same time had guilt, self-mutilation fantasies, and was paranoid. The manic state can have these variations from the standard typical mania (DSM-IV-TR™ 2000, pp. 413–14).

These symptoms had been controlled by medication—clozapine, high doses of sertraline (Zoloft), clonazepam (Klonopin), and valproic acid (Depakote), but she was still left with some characterologic symptoms, e.g., excessive sensitivity in interpersonal relations with a "chip on the shoulder" when she talked with people. She tried to learn tact, at first with some difficulty, but later very well. She also had considerable anxiety clinically so that she had to use clonazepam regularly when under stress. Although these symptoms existed, there has been the saving virtue of being able to relate to the therapist and hear the suggestions and interpretations and try to put them into practice. This effective therapeutic alliance was there and working throughout the entire illness. In any less intensive therapy without an empathic relationship this might not be possible. She formerly spent her spare time with a closed group of sometimes hospitalized people who were disabled for work, went to group meetings, and were supported by families or Medicare; but she was now able to function satisfactorily in the college atmosphere and was accepted readily by the college-age group. In fact, she was respected and looked up to, which gave her a grasp of herself as a respected, more active person. The new adult self is emerging.

In the use of multiple systems in the process of therapy, this method resembles the Multi-System Therapy described for treating delinquent adolescents, and the Personal Therapy used for the treatment of schizophrenics (Fenton 1997) and the Cognitive Behavioral analysis system described by McCullough (2000). However, in detail the therapy included long-range work with all the issues contributing to the predicament.

This case is an example of a typically difficult case with the complication that once the *symptoms* of the illness are controlled it is necessary and possible to attempt to treat the *functional impairments*. These impairments were: (1) a comorbid anxiety state with phobias, and (2) a characterologic disorder of paranoid and schizoid type in a person who had never really matured. Each of these two impairments required specific treatment. When the psychosis was

179

brought under control it became possible to treat the phobias, and concurrently the character defects, as follows:

1. Treatment of comorbid anxieties, e.g., phobias. She had an elevator phobia, not wanting to use an elevator when someone else was in it or might get on with her. When she and the analyst therapist decided to work on this phobia, she remembered that during her therapy in late adolescence she had had a brief period when the same phobia occurred. It came to the surface as she discussed this phobia with her analyst at that time that she was afraid of being attacked sexually if on an elevator with a man, and her awakening sexual feelings were involved. The phobia lessened enough after this revelation that when she bravely took elevators as a trial she was able to do it, and the lingering fantasy gradually became just a passing thought.

2. Treatment of low self-image. In the third phase of her treatment, she began to work on her vulnerability to slights and the tendency to fantasize attacks and insults when none were made. The fear of failure in classes became less and less as she was successful in the courses she took in school. Her decision not to take a full schedule made sense as she had been out of school a long time and was not confident in her ability to do the work. She was able gradually

to assert herself with her family and take a firmer attitude toward speaking up in family situations. She spent more time working at her studies and stopped just sitting around the coffee house with the group of disabled persons.

3. As to the question of diagnosis, the subject of psychotic depression is somewhat uncertain nowadays. No longer is it confined to what used to be called involutional melancholia. Since the recognition of a cycling illness with some schizoid-paranoid symptoms called schizoaffective and the disappearance of hysterical psychosis, it seems more appropriate to call the patient schizoaffective, bipolar type.

Summary of the Case

This patient had had intensive psychodynamic therapy for several years as an adolescent and was able to use the insights gained in that therapy once the psychosis was controlled by medication. However, during the period of several years of therapy and getting the psychosis under control, she did not have as intensive insight therapy as psychoanalysis allows, as the first chronic patient described in this chapter had received. That first patient was able to work through her very traumatic childhood fixations and traumas and acquire a new "self." It did not seem possible or necessary or even feasible to attack this second patient's problem with a classical psychoanalysis. Psychoanalysis was given serious consideration and a battle with Medicare was considered also, but progress was constantly being interrupted by breakdowns until clozapine was started. Once that medication was started, progress continued in a satisfactory way so that analysis did not seem necessary.

However, because she had previously (in adolescence) received analytic psychotherapy for several years, it was possible in once- or twice-weekly hourly visits to use enough psychodynamic therapy for her to grow and mature and also acquire a healthier adult "self." A healthier "self" means a better and stronger personality, giving a better balance and a lesser negative score on the "predicament" equation. In addition, on the positive side, she had asked to have a woman therapist in place of the man who was to retire. Like so many other patients with mood disorders, the "important other" continues to be important even when the personality becomes stronger with therapy and growth. By having a woman therapist, she would acquire many feminine features in her new adult "self." From the outset, she had a consistent ability to form a very effective therapeutic alliance, which was there through thick and thin.

In contrast to the sicker patients with serious personality disorders and more severe illnesses, like this patient, there are others who have been able to handle their illness with less intensive psychotherapy, because of less severe illness plus a much healthier personality with a good deal of strength. For example, the widow who raised three children and held a responsible job when her depressions were brought under control with medication. Another example is a man employed by an international corporation who has been able to travel the world in his work and handle a very heavy load of responsibility. Both of these patients would have very good scores on the predicament equation.

In closing, I would emphasize that the common denominators with all patients are an interested and involved physician who is able to form an effective doctor-patient relationship and a patient who is able to form an effective therapeutic alliance. This combination creates a method of introducing into the patient's life a person who can substitute for the important other, whatever contribution is needed to help the patient develop and strengthen his personality and manage his life. This relationship is in addition to making sure that the patient gets the best medical treatment currently available. Also, strengthening of the personality by overcoming long-standing deficits through psychoanalysis is something that medicines alone would not accomplish. In some cases, medication relieves some long-standing symptoms that look like personality characteristics. If medicine relieves them, I prefer to regard the relieved symptoms as part of the depression. If they are not relieved by medicine, I prefer to consider them as personality symptoms and recommend intensive, long-term psychodynamic and/or thorough insight therapy, whichever is appropriate, including psychoanalysis in some cases.

8
Summary and Conclusions

CHAPTER-BY-CHAPTER SUMMARY

The following chapter-by-chapter summary of the entire book is presented to enable the reader to find a particular subject in detail.

The purpose of this book is first to formulate a method for identifying the predicament that is the cause of chronicity and then to formulate specific methods of treating those chronic cases, especially those that have appeared refractory, i.e., treatment resistant.

There are two parts to the book. In Part I, the concept of a "predicament" is defined and its role identified as the basis of the chronicity of the symptoms. Chronicity, treatment resistance, and refractory mood disorders are defined and causes identified and listed. The frequency of chronic cases is noted to be at least in the 25- to 35-percent range, using the observations of the author's practice with 10- and 25-year follow-up as about 35 to 40 percent of the initial cases. These numbers are confirmed by examinations of the considerable literature in recent years. Treatment is discussed in Part II.

The predicament is described in detail in case examples, and listed as caused by the existence of stressful factors enumerated according to the method of the 5 axes of the Multiaxial System of the *Diagnostic and Statistical Manual IV*. A scoring system using numbers 1 to 10 indicates the severity of each factor and then adds the numbers, giving a total of the negatives. This is balanced against the positive items to give a final number by which the patient is scored as potentially either chronic because of a predicament, borderline chronic, or not likely to be chronic.

In Chapter 1, a method of identifying the cause of the chronicity is described. The cause is called, for practical purposes, a "predicament," and it is described as being present in patients who are refractory to the initial treatment. Based on clinical observations made by the author, the original description of the predicament stated that it was caused by a combination of 2 factors: (1) an intolerably painful and troublesome relationship with the partner of the patient, whom we call the "important other," and (2) a personality deficit that prevented the patient from solving that relationship problem in an acceptable and tolerable way. Thus the situation became chronic and

186

persistent, and the depression became persistent and chronic.

In Chapter 2, the current definition of chronicity, refractory, and treatment-resistant mood disorders is given, as it is now accepted in the field and stated in the literature. It is emphasized that refractory refers to those cases that do not respond acceptably to the standard currently accepted today and does not refer to patients who are noncompliant or inadequately treated according to present-day standards.

Chapter 3 describes the occurrence of chronicity in 25- and 10-year follow–ups of cases seen in the author's practice, typically 35 to 40 percent of the initial cases. Of the patients seen 25 years earlier, a total of 38 cases were mood disorders, of whom 37 percent were known to be chronic by definition, and 20 percent are still in contact and on medication. Twenty-six percent of the 49 patients with mood disorders seen 10 years ago are still in contact, and there may be more chronic patients in the group who were not followed by the author.

Chapter 4 explores the question of chronicity as reported in the literature. The report of the Pittsburgh group (Kupfer 1995) showing that discontinuing the medication after symptomatic recovery from the initial attack of depression resulted in eventual recurrences became the accepted standard for continuing medication indefinitely because of chronicity of the tendency to depression. As stated by Judd (1999), "There is an increasing realization that unipolar major depressive disorder (MDD) is primarily a chronic disease." Several new concepts have arisen: the concept of chronicity, treatment resistance and its causes, an underlying core process, functioning beyond acute symptoms, comorbidity, and the importance of the doctor-patient relationship.

Chapter 5 describes a numerical method of using the Multiaxial System to score the patient as to the potential for chronicity and for becoming refractory. Of course, clinical judgment is never to be abandoned and the score may not be the final answer, but a high negative score showing the potentially troublesome factors should alert the clinician to the potential for treatment resistance and help him or her to be on the lookout for it. Actually, if the physician has been alert and careful enough to observe the potentially troublesome factors as listed on the Multiaxial System, that observation in itself makes therapy possible.

In Part II, Chapters 6 and 7, the specialized methods of treatment are described. One method stated by Weissman (1999, p. 220) is to look beyond the core biological symptoms of mood and vegetative signs and examine drive, motivation, performance, and quality of interpersonal relations that are not captured on the traditional symptom scales. It must also be emphasized that standard initial treatment with medication, counseling, attention to the various stresses, etc., is to be prescribed and acted upon first. The chronicity and its causes in symptoms and personality require special consideration and special attitudes on the part of the therapist. Treatment is thus directed to both symptoms and causes.

Chapter 6 takes up the principles of treatment and the methods needed for this group of patients. The doctor-patient relationship is described in detail as a special therapeutic device, a therapeutic alliance. It is especially important with this group of patients, who take more time than the simpler cases, thus allowing the relationship to develop. Pharmacotherapy is emphasized but is not described in detail—it is left to specialized contributions (see Appendix I to identify specific medications current at the time of this writing). The type of intervention requiring management and counseling is described also. Various types of psychotherapy, including cognitive, behavioral, interpersonal, psychodynamic, and psychoanalytic therapy and its derivatives, are described; and case examples are given to illustrate the flexible and combined methods required with this group of patients. Combined methods are tailored to the individual need. The phases of treatment are given in detail—acute, continuation, and maintenance plus rehabilitation as needed.

In Chapter 7, the use of combinations of pharmacotherapy, psychotherapy, and other psychosocial therapies is described. The phases of treatment from symptom relief, to rehabilitation, back to the functioning mainstream population are illustrated with examples. The first example is a bipolar I patient who had a 6-year, 5-session-a-week psychoanalysis, in and out of the hospital, with some electroconvulsant therapy also when she was at her worst. This patient is described to give an illustration of the childhood origin of characterologic symptoms in the experiencing of trauma, losses, and sexual overstimulation. The case study illustrates how the patient's analysis helped her to get back into a normal marriage and a healthy motherhood. It serves as an example of the many cases of mood-disorder patients seen by the author who were enormously helped by psychoanalysis or its derivatives—psychodynamic psychotherapy. Another successful patient with a bipolar schizoaffective disorder is described in detail, illustrating the use of modern psychopharmacology with an atypical antipsychotic, clozapine, combined with an antidepressant and a mood leveler. This medication allowed the patient to receive intensive, insight-oriented psychotherapy for several years and become rehabilitated after many years of illness, in and out of hospitals. She was helped enormously by having had 5 years of psychoanalytic psychotherapy in adolescence. The process of rehabilitation is described as the ultimate goal of therapy of the chronic patients, and is illustrated by examples. In summary, where personality defect is part of the cause of chronicity of the depression, i.e., of the predicament, the psychodynamic-psychoanalytic method is useful in treatment and can modify and actually cure these defects, thus solving the predicament.

CONCLUSIONS

More than 20 years ago, I recognized that depressions frequently became chronic when certain circumstances existed in the patient's life: namely the presence of what I defined *a predicament*—a very stressful circum-stance—coupled with a personality problem that pre-vented the patient from solving the problem. My practice over the last 20-plus years and the experience of others in the field have supported that observation and have enabled me to expand on the concept of the predicament and develop some guidelines for its iden-tification and treatment.

Almost any mood disorder can be chronic and/or refractory, and a large proportion of patients with mood disorders fall into this category (40 to 70 percent in various recent studies). I have presented an analysis of patients with mood disorders for my 55 years of practice, looking at the status in the year 2000 of patients in treatment for 10 years and for 25 years. This review of cases showed that a large proportion of patients in private practice is chronically ill and will require long-term treatment to get well. The analysis further showed that this treatment must in-clude identification and treatment of the psychosocial problems in terms of the meaning of the situation to the patient and his or her personality. Also, the review suggested that psychoanalytic therapy and its deriva-tives are very helpful in bringing about improvements in functioning, especially for long-standing personal-ity problems.

A number of concepts have contributed to the development of the guidelines presented in this book. The concept that mood disorders are potentially chronic illnesses and must be treated as such is a relatively new one to some workers in the field. Also, it is now recognized that some patients do not respond well to medication, that in each case there is a common underlying cause that should be identified, that the functioning of the patient must be taken into account, that the doctor-patient relationship is especially important in treatment of chronic mood disorders, and that comorbidity is commonly a cause of treatment resistance.

Using information from my practice and results of published studies, I revised my description of the predicament to include 16 factors, related these factors to the 5 categories of the DSM-IV, and created a scoring scheme. Also, I recognized that some factors serve to help the patient solve the predicament and so reduce the likelihood of the illness becoming chronic. I identified 5 such factors, which I call positive factors. I have illustrated the application of this diagnostic method with case examples from my own practice.

I then turn to treatment of chronic mood disorders and point out that both relief of symptoms and functional recovery are the goals of treatment. I outline individual treatment techniques that are currently available and then discuss the use of combined schools of psychotherapy treatment techniques. Although the introduction of effective medication has helped many patients with mood disorders, it has become clear that in many cases, medication alone does not cure the patient. Some mood-disorder patients respond well to one treatment method, but in most cases a combination of psychotherapeutic methods is required.

Treatment is now considered to have three phases: acute, continuation, and maintenance. Although these are not completely distinct from each other, the recognition of these phases is a useful guideline to assess the patient's progress to the fourth phase, rehabilitation.

I end the book with detailed case presentations to illustrate the kind of detailed work the therapist has to be prepared to do. These cases illustrate the application of the Multiaxial System described, the phases of treatment, and the response.

The major conclusions that I would like the reader to draw from this book are:

1. Depressive illness very often becomes chronic, recurrent, or recovers only partially. Even with acceptable standard present-day, conventional, short-term treatment (up to 2 years), many patients with mood disorders do not get completely "well." Being "well" means not only with symptom relief but also functioning normally. If not functioning well despite some symptom relief, the patient can be considered chronic.

2. Most of these chronically ill patients can be identified by careful examination and are characterized by what I call a "predicament." This consists of a combination of a highly unsatisfactory living situation, usually concerning the relationship with the partner or the most important other person, or the absence of a caring person, plus a personality problem that pre-

193

vents the patient from solving the living problem in a satisfactory way.

3. Long-term combined therapy, continued appropriate medication, and more frequent and intensive sessions than the standard short-term treatment are needed and can clear up the unsatisfactory situation, relieve symptoms, and bring about a return to normal function.

4. The doctor-patient relationship must become a long-term therapeutic alliance between the patient and the therapist, with sufficiently intensive, appropriate psychotherapy to resolve the psychological personal issues in the predicament. This is done by doing two things—one, by uncovering and resolving the identifiable factors in the patient's life that caused the predicament, and two, by treating the personality problems.

5. Systematic evaluation of the patient's situation using the Multiaxial System of the *Diagnostic and Statistical Manual* helps the doctor recognize the chronic mood disorders and the personal issues contributing to the predicament, and helps the doctor design treatment.

6. Combined treatment—i.e., medication, psychosocial intervention, psychotherapy (sometimes intensive), plus rehabilitation—is commonly

required for patients with chronic mood disorders. There has to be a very involved and always-available professional who "cares"—the therapist, a case manager, or a psychiatrist—who sees that all these treatment programs get done. Because of the complexity of both current psychopharmacology and effective psychotherapy, it is difficult for one person to be sufficiently expert to handle both fields. As a result, nowadays it is common for the patient to be treated medically by a physician, usually a psychiatrist who knows the drugs, and also by a psychotherapist trained to perform the advanced kind of psychotherapy needed in the chronic cases. This collaborative program, currently known as "split treatment," requires knowledgeable communication and cooperation by both persons (see Fawcett 1994).

7. The personality problems may require intensive psychodynamic treatment or psychoanalysis to correct long-standing character problems and to allow the patient to catch up for lost time.

8. The appropriate use of medication usually makes a successful psychotherapy workable.

In closing, I hope these pages provide both a flexible clinical method of combining the two sciences—

biological and psychological—to identify the problems creating the predicament in chronic patients and provide a comprehensive method of treating these problems to successfully bring the patients back into the mainstream of life.

Annotated Reference List

A Recovering Patient.* (1986). "Can we talk?" The schizophrenic patient in psychotherapy. *American Journal of Psychiatry* 143: 68–70.

———. (1998). Medication-psychotherapy combination most effective for schizophrenia. *Psychiatric Times Monograph* 28:30.

Acocella, J. (2000). The empty couch: what is left when psychiatry turns to drugs? *The New Yorker* May 8, pp. 82–88.

Akil, H., and Watson, S. J. (2000). Science and the future of psychiatry. *Archives of General Psychiatry* 57:86–87.

American Psychiatric Association. *Diagnostic and Sta-*

*To maintain confidentiality the patient's name is withheld.

tistical Manual of Mental Disorders (2000). 4th ed., Text Revision (DSM–IV TR™). Washington, D.C.

Angst, Jules. (1992). How recurrent and predictable is depressive illness? In *Long-Term Treatment of Depression, Perspectives in Psychiatry,* vol. 3, ed. S. A. Montgomery and F. Rauillon. Guildford, England: John Wiley & Sons.

Badal, D. W. (1968). Transitional and pre-psychotic symptoms in depression. *Bulletin of the Philadelphia Psychoanalytic Association* 15:10–25.

———. (1979). Eclectic therapy in difficult depressions. *Proceedings of the Annual Meeting of the American Psychiatric Association,* May 18, p. 367.

———. (1981). Chronic disability in depressive disorders—the influence of psychological factors. Paper Presented at Annual Meeting of American Psychiatric Association.

———. (1988). *Treatment of Depression and Related Moods.* Northvale, New Jersey. New Orleans, May 1981.

———. (2000). Mourning or melancholia—a diagnostic dilemma. *Child Analysis* 11:141–168.

Berlanga, Carlos, et al. (1999). Personality and clinical predictors of recurrence of depression. *Psychiatric Services* 50(3): 376–380.

Berman, R. M., Narisimhan, Meera, and Charney, D. S. (1997). Treatment-refractory depression: definitions and characteristics. *Depression and Anxiety* 5:154–164.

Bird, Brian. (1973). *Talking with Patients.* 2nd ed. Philadelphia: J. B. Lippincott.

Blum, H. P. (1999). The reconstruction of reminiscence. *Journal of the American Psychoanalytic Association* 47:1125–43.

> p. 1125: "The process of reconstruction integrates and transcends memory, facilitating personality reorganization."

Bowlby, J. (1969). *Attachment and Loss*. London: Hogarth Press.

———. (1988) Developmental psychiatry comes of age. *American Journal of Psychiatry* 145(1):1–10.

Cassidy, Jude, and Shaver, Phillip R., eds. (1999). *Handbook of Attachment: Theory, Research, and Clinical Applications*. New York: Guilford Press.

Ciechanowski, P. S., et al. (2001). The patient-provider relationship: attachment theory and adherence to treatment in diabetes. *American Journal of Psychiatry* 158(1): 29–35.

Commission on Professional and Hospital Activities. *International Classification of Diseases, 9th Revision, Clinical Modification* (ICD-9-CM) (2001). Ann Arbor, MI.

Delgado, Pedro L. (2000). Depression: The Case for a Monoamine Deficiency. *Jour. Clinical Psychiatry:* 2000; 61 (supplement 6, pp. 7–11. The complexity of the neurochemical changes involved in depression is explained in this paper reporting studies involving the influence of monoamine depletion on the effect of antidepressant treatment. He states the following: "In conclusion, it is clear that antidepressant agents in current use do indeed

require intact monoamine systems for their therapeutic effect." (p. 7). He adds, "However, some
debate remains as to the precise role that a deficiency in monoamine system(s) may play in depression itself."

———. (2001). Neurotransmitters affect the efficacy
of antidepressants. In American Psychiatric Association Symposia Highlights on the Treatment of
Depressive Disorders. *Psychiatric Annals, Supplement*. Thorofare, NH. Charles Lack.

A very helpful and specific clinical guide, based on
neurophysiological principles and describing the
use of specific antidepressants for specific symptoms. A must read for the person treating the
patient.

Delgado's paper includes a graph illustrating the
specific symptoms affected by (1) the serotonin
mechanism, (2) the norepinephrine, and (3) both.
The table below summarizes his graph.

Serotonin	Norepinephrine	Both
Impulsivity	Motivation	Mood
Sexual Function	Energy, Interest	Sleep
Appetite	Concentration	Anxiety
		Stress
		Coping

Fawcett, Jan. (1994). Progress in treatment-resistant and treatment-refractory depression: we still have a long way to go. *Journal of Clinical Psychiatry* 24:214–216.

———. (2001). An issue that must be addressed. *Psychiatric Annals* 31(10):582.

Fenton, W. S., et al. (1997). Symptom subtype and suicidality in patients with schizophrenic spectrum disorders. *American Journal of Psychiatry* 154(2):199–204.

Feske, Ulrike, et al. (2000). Anxiety as a correlate of response to the acute treatment of bipolar I disorder. *American Journal of Psychiatry* 157: 956–962.

Anxiety predicts a poor outcome in the acute treatment of bipolar disorder.

Frank, Ellen, and Kupfer, D. J. (2000). Peeking through the door at the 21st century. *Archives of General Psychiatry* 57:81–83.

How does life experience alter gene expression in vulnerable individuals? What are the neurobiological effects of psychotherapy?

Freud, A. (1971). Letter. *American Journal of Psychiatry* 140:1583.

Greenson, R. R. (1967). *The Technique and Practice of Psychoanalysis*, vol. 1, pp. 151–357. New York: International Universities Press.

Hamilton, M. (1960). A rating scale for depression. *Journal of Neurology, Neurosurgery and Psychiatry* 25:56–62.

Harvard Medical School. (2000). Antisocial personality disorder, part I. *Harvard Mental Health Letter* 17(6):Dec. p. 1.

Haykal R. F. and Akiskal, H. S. (1999). The long-term outcome of dysthymia in private practice: clinical features, temperament, and the art of management. *Journal of Clinical Psychiatry* 60:508–518.

Hirschfeld, R.M.A. (2001). Bipolar spectrum disorder: improving its recognition and diagnosis. *Journal of Clinical Psychiatry* 62 (Supplement 14):5–9.

Hyman, S. E. (2000). The millenium of mind, brain, and behavior. *Archives of General Psychiatry* 57: 88–89.

Judd, L. L. (1999). Treatment-resistant depression: guidelines for early diagnosis and recognition. *Proceedings of the Annual Meeting of the American Psychiatric Association*, p. 223. Washington, D.C.: American Psychiatric Association.

There are three major goals in the treatment of major depressive episodes: (1) removal of depressive symptoms; (2) reduction or elimination of the associated impairment; and (3) the prevention of episode relapse or recurrence. Failure to achieve any or all of these treatment goals should be used to define treatment-resistant depression (TRD).

Judd, L. L., Paulus, M. P., and Zeller, P. (1999). The role of residual subthreshold depressive symptoms in early episode relapse in unipolar major depressive disorder. *Archives of General Psychiatry* 56(8):764–765.

Judd, L. L., et al. (2000). Psychosocial disability during the long-term course of unipolar major depressive disorder. *Archives of General Psychiatry* 57:375 (abstract).

Kandel, E. R. (1999a). Biology and the future of psychoanalysis: a new intellectual framework for psychiatry revisited. *American Journal of Psychiatry* 156:505–524.

———. (1999b). Dr. Kandel replies. *American Journal of Psychiatry* 158(4):665.

———. (2001). Nobel prize winner to speak at annual meeting. *Psychiatric News*, May 4, p. 1849.

Klein, D. W., et al. (2000). Five-year course and outcome of dysthymic disorder; a prospective, naturalistic follow-up study. *American Journal of Psychiatry* 157(6):931–939.

Kraepelin, Emil. (1921). *Manic-Depressive Insanity and Paranoia*. Edinburgh: E. & S. Livingston.

The classic. Describes in impressive detail the symptoms and the several different courses that manic-depressive disease (now "bipolar disorder") can take. Also, separates out the classical paranoid from the other psychotic conditions.

Krueger, R. F. (1999). The structure of common mental disorders. *Archives of General Psychiatry* 56:921–926.

Krueger concludes: "The results offer a novel perspective on comorbidity, suggesting the comorbidity results from common, underlying core psychopathological processes. The results thereby argue for focusing research on these core processes themselves, rather than on their varied manifestations as separate disorders."

Kupfer, D. J. (1995). Acute continuation and maintenance treatment of mood disorders. *Depression* 3:137–138.

The phases of treatment are: acute, continuation, and maintenance. Most individuals will suffer recurrences, suggesting a need to develop long-term strategies. The continuation phase should last approximately 20 weeks if symptoms have remained in remission or recovery status has been reached. New studies show that medication should be continued at the same dose as in the acute phase, and also throughout the maintenance phase (what gets you well keeps you well). Recently specific forms of psychotherapy have shown considerable efficacy not only for shortterm treatments but also over the long term. We need to focus increasing attention on the adaptation of shortterm treatment for the long term. Research is needed on combination treatments in both unipolar and bipolar disorders.

Kupfer, D. J. and Frank, Ellen. (1992). The minimum length of treatment for recovery. In *Perspectives in*

Psychiatry, vol. 1: Long Term Treatment of Depression. Chichester, England: John Wiley and Sons.

————. (1997). Role of psychosocial factors in the onset of major depression. *Annals of the New York Academy of Sciences* 807:429–439.

Loeb, F. F. and Loeb, L. R. (1987). The effect of pharmacotherapy on manic attacks. *Journal of the American Psychoanalytic Association* 35:877–902.

Mazer, M. (1976) People and Predicaments. *Harvard University Press.*

Mazure, C. M. et al. (2000). Adverse life events and cognitive-personality characteristics in the prediction of major depression and antidepressant response. *American Journal of Psychiatry* 157:896–903.

McCullough, J. P., Jr. (2000). *Treatment for Chronic Depression:Cognitive Behavioral Analysis System of Psychotherapy*. New York: Guilford Press.

A very successful process in the treatment of chronic depression. However, it is so structured that a well-trained therapist would not need it. The method of analyzing the transference could help to treat interpersonal symptoms.

Miller, M. C. (2001). Attachment and the therapeutic relationship. *Harvard Mental Health Letter*. May, pp. 7–8.

Montgomery, S. A., and Asberg, M. (1979). A new depression scale designed to be sensitive to change. *British Journal of Psychiatry* 134:382–389.

National Depressive and Manic-Depressive Association. *Beyond Diagnosis: A Landmark Survey on Depression and its Treatment.* Chicago: The National Depressive and Manic-Depressive Association. 2000.

Nemeroff, C. B. (1998). The neurobiology of depression. *Scientific American,* June 1998, pp. 42–47.

> My colleagues and I propose that early abuse or neglect not only activates the stress response but induces persistently increased activity in CRG-containing neurons, which are known to be stress responsive and to be over-active in depressed people. If the hyperactivity in the neurons of children persisted through adulthood, these supersensitive cells would react vigorously even to mild stresses. This effect in people already innately predisposed to depression could then produce both the neuroendocrine and behavioral responses characteristic of the disorder.

Nesse, R. M. (2000). Is depression an adaptation? *Archives of General Psychiatry* 57(1): 14–20.

Oates, J. C. (2001). I'm not O.K., you're not O.K. A personal account of one man's battle against chronic depression (review). *New York Times Book Review,* p. 9. June 24, 2001.

O'Reardon, J. P., and Amsterdam, J. D. (1998). Treatment-resistant depression: progress and limitation. *Psychiatric Annals* 28 (11):633–640.

Price, J. S. (1978). Chronic depressive illness. *British Medical Journal* 1 (6121):1200–1201.

Ritsner, Michael, et al. (2000). Differences in quality of life domains and psychopathologic and psychosocial factors in psychiatric patients. *Journal of Clinical Psychiatry* 61:880–889.

> P. 880: "Psychosocial factors rather that psychopathologic symptoms affect QOL (quality of life) of hospitalized patients with severe mental disorders. The findings enable better understanding of the combining effects of psychopathologic and psychosocial factors on subjective life satisfaction and highlight targets for more effective intervention and rehabilitation."

Rogers, W. H., et al. (1993). Outcomes for adult outpatients with depression under prepaid or fee-for-service financing. *Archives of General Psychiatry* 50(7):517–525.

Rush, A. J., and Thase, M. E. (1997). Strategies and tactics in the treatment of chronic depression. *Journal of Clinical Psychiatry* 58 (Supplement 13): 14–22.

A good definition of chronicity:

> "Chronic depressions include major depressive disorder, recurrent, without full inter-episode recovery; major depressive disorder, currently in a chronic (i.e., > 2

years) episode; double depression; dysthymic disorder, and those depressive disorders—not otherwise specified (NOS)—that are persistent or predictably recurrent with substantial disability." They raise substantial questions about the treatment of these chronic illnesses. In this book I will try to give a general system of approach that I hope will allow us to study methods of treatment systematically, namely, to separate treatment into phases that can be separated out and studied as to methods of treatment.

Sadek, Noha, and Bona, Joseph. (2000). Subsyndromal symptomatic depression: a new concept. *Depression and Anxiety* 12(1):30–39.

An excellent review of the kind of common depression that is of great importance in practice and recently has received a good deal of attention in research. A thorough review of references.

"The high prevalence of SSD, the significant psychosocial impairment associated with it, and the chronicity of its course makes subsyndromal subsymptomatic depressions a matter for serious consideration by clinicians and researchers."

Sajatovic, M., and Mullen, J. A. (1999). *Manual of Rating Scales for the Assessment of Serious Mental Illness*. Wilmington, DE: AstraZeneca.

Sartorius, N. (2001). The economic and social burden of depression. *Journal of Clinical Psychiatry* 62 (Supplement 15):8–11.

Schore, N. A. (1994). *Affect Regulation and the Origin of Self: Neurology of Emotional Development*. Hillsdale, NJ: Lawrence Erlbaum and Associates.

Soloff, P. H. (1998). Algorithms for pharmacological treatment of personality dimensions: symptom-specific treatments for cognitive-perceptual, affective, and impulsive-behavioral dysregulation. *Bulletin of the Menninger Clinic* 62(2):195–214.

Stroh, Michael. (1999). Doctors make house calls: online "clinics," physicians are changing the face of medicine. *Cleveland Plain Dealer*, July 12, p. 1F.

Swindle, R. W. et al. (1998). Risk factors for sustained non-remission of depressive symptoms. *Journal of Nervous and Mental Disease* 186:462–469.

In a study of 370 patients with unipolar depressive disorder, four years after initial treatment 43 percent had significant depressive symptoms. Factors that predicted the chronic course were: less education, or more severe initial depressive mood and ideation, secondary major depression, prior treatment, comorbid medical conditions, and fewer close relationships, as well as serious medical conditions. Acute stressful life events, marital status, and age did not predict the chronic course.

Tasman, A. (2000). Presidential address: the doctor-patient relationship. *American Journal of Psychiatry* 157(11):1762–68.

Thase, M. E., Friedman, E. S., and Howland, R. H. (2001). Is depression-focused psychotherapy just an elaborate placebo? *The Economics of Neuroscience*. August: 52–61.

Weissman, M. M. (1997). Beyond symptoms: social functioning and the new antidepressants. *Journal of Psychopharmacology* 11 (supplement): S5–S8.

———. (1999). Social functioning with the new treatments for depression. *American Psychiatric Association, Proceedings of the Annual Meeting* No. 3E, p. 221. Washington, DC; American Psychiatric Association.

Depression scales assess the core biological features of the illness—mood, pessimism, and vegetative signs, (e.g., appetite and sleep loss). However, assessments of drive, motivation, performance, and quality of interpersonal relations (e.g., the social context once the symptoms are improved) may not be captured in the traditional symptom scales. There is often a need for further treatment when the basic symptoms are controlled.

Wittchen, H-U., Hofler, Michael, and Merikangas, Kathleen. (1999). Toward the identification of core psychopathological processes? *Archives of General Psychiatry* 56:929–931.

Wylie, H. W., Jr. and Wylie, M. L. (1987). An effect of pharmacotherapy on the psychoanalytic process: case report of a modified analysis. *American Journal of Psychiatry* 144: 489–492.

Zisook, Sidney, Shuchter, S. R., and Dunn, L. B. (2001). Grief and depression: diagnostic and treatment challenges. *Primary Psychiatry* 8(5):37–53.
Zung. W. W. (1965). A self-rating depression scale. *Archives of General Psychiatry* 12: 63–70.

Appendix I
Medications Currently Used
for Treatment of Mood Disorders

P hase I is the usual time that medication is started, but in any phase—I, II, or III—it may have to be changed. Tables A1–A8 list medications used and the symptoms for which they are prescribed. Table A1 lists medications used as antidepressants; A2 those used as anti-anxiety medications; A3 the neuroleptic and antipsychotic medications; A4 the benzodiazepine and the non-benzodiazepine hypnotic medications; A5 the antimanic and the antimanic, anticonvulsant medications; and A6 the antipsychotic medications.

Combinations of medications have been found to be useful at times, since the two or three drugs augment the beneficial effect of one another.

Table A1.   Antidepressant medications in current and frequent use.

Generic Name	Brand Name(s)
Tricyclics	
Amitriptyline hydrochloride	Amitril, Elavil, Endep
Clomipramine hydrochloride	Anafranil
Imipramine hydrochloride	Tofranil
Selective Serotonin Reuptake Inhibitors	
Citalopram	Celexa
Fluoxetine hydrochloride	Prozac
Fluoxamine maleate	Luvox
Paroxetine hydrochloride	Paxil
Sertraline hydrochloride	Zoloft
Selective Serotonin-Norepinephrine Reuptake Inhibitors	
Venlafaxin hydrochloride	Effexor (XR)
Atypical Antidepressants	
Bupropion hydrochloride	Wellbutrin
Mirtazepine	Remeron
5-HT2 Antagonists	
Nefazodone hydrochloride	Serzone
Trazodone hydrochloride	Desyrel

Table A2. Anti-anxiety medications in current and frequent use.

Generic	Brand Name
Benzodiazepines	
Alprazolam	Xanax
Chlordiazepoxide hydrochloride	Librium and others
Clonazepam	Klonopin
Clorazepate dipotassium	Tranxene
Diazepam	Valium
Halazepam	Paxipam
Lorazepam	Ativan
Oxazepam	Serax
Prazepam	Centrax
Antihistamines	
Diphenhydramine	Benadryl
Hydroxyzine hydrochloride	Atarax, Vistaril

Table A3. Anti-obsessive-compulsive-disorder medications in current and frequent use.

Generic	Brand Name
Clomipramine hydrochloride	Anafranil
Fluvoxamine maleate	Luvox

Table A4. Hypnotic medications in current and frequent use.

Generic	Brand Name
Benzodiazepine hypnotics	
Estazolam	ProSom
Flurazepam hydrochloride	Dalmane
Quazepam	Doral
Temazepam	Restoril
Triazolam	Halcion
Non-Benzodiazepine Hypnotics	
Chloral hydrate	Noctex
Diphenhydramine HCL	Benadryl
Zolpidem tartrate	Ambien

Table A5. Antimanic medications in current and frequent use.

Generic	Brand Name
Antimanic; lithium compounds, mostly salts	
Lithium carbonate	Eskalith, Lithane, LITHOBID, LITHOTABS
Lithium citrate	Citrailith
Verapamil hydrochloride	Calan
Antimanic, Anticonvulsant	
Carbamazepine	Tegretol
Gabapentin	Neurontin
Lamotrigine	Lamictal
Valproic acid	Depakene, Depakote

Table A6. Antipsychotic medications in current and frequent use.

Generic	Brand Name
Benzisoxazole derivatives	
Risperidone	Risperdal—atypical
Butyrophenones	
Haloperidol	Haldol
Dibenzodiazepines	
Clozapine	Clozaril—atypical
Loxapine hydrochloride	Loxitane
Dibenzothiazepines	
Quetiapine	Seroquel—atypical
Thioxanthenes	
Thiothixene	Navane
Dehydroindolone	
Molindone hydrochloride	Moban
Diphenylbutylpiperidine	
Pimozide	Orap
Phenothiazine, aliphatic	
Chlopromazine	Thorazine
Phenothiazine, piperazine	
Fluphenazine	Prolixin
Perphenazine	Trilafon, Etrafon
Thioridazine	Mellaril
Thienobenzodiazepine	
Olanzepine	Zyprexa—atypical
Ziprasidone	Geodon—atypical

Appendix II
Example of Documentation for Gaining Approval for a Program of Rehabilitation of a Patient with a Chronic Mood Disorder

These two letters to the patient's insurance company tell the story of the launching of a rehabilitation program for a patient with chronic depression. This is a brief example of what it is like to get a rehabilitation program underway, when it is feasible to do it with a chronic patient, and when it is likely to succeed. The reader will be interested to know that the program continues to be successful. However, the time involved in the communication with the insurance company is not reimbursed, and the company reimburses for the office visits at the rate of 50 percent of the allowed fee, so one has to have a certain amount of dedication to do this work for a living because typically the patient is not able to make up the difference. Co-payment by the patient is not allowed in certain contracts, but many patients will make up the difference if the contract is explained to them as optional.

Some public clinics have begun to employ the personnel to do the job correctly. One has to search around to find a clinic that can give enough intensive psychotherapy as well as the expertise in the up-to-date use of medication. This is another example of "split treatment"—in a clinic of professionals who have the expertise and knowledge to work together, good results may be obtained.

FIRST REQUEST:

DATE:

TO: The patient's insurance company

Re: John Doe (the patient)

Dear Administrator:

This is to supplement the authorization form enclosed to explain more clearly why we need more treatment sessions with the above-named John Doe, your client of many years.

There is a history of several psychiatric hospitalizations starting in 1980, and treatment with ECT. Since that time, he has been chronically disabled, with major depression and a chronic pain condition.

However, in the last two years under therapy with his counselor he has embarked on an attempt to overcome his disability, as follows:

1. An intensive chronic pain treatment program at the hospital here, starting in January of this year. He has shown 50 percent improvement, and completed the program this month.

2. Enrollment in March 2001 with the Bureau of Vocational Disability, for the possibility of training for work within his physical limits, such as deskwork with computers.

3. Intensive psychotherapy with his counselor-therapist (named Rev. Richard Roe) has helped to lower serious personal stresses at home that threatened to interfere with recovery. This should continue at a twice-weekly pace.

4. Beginning of a modern psychopharmacotherapy treatment with me to relieve a very serious major depression and anxiety with phobias, obsessions, and compulsions. This should continue with once-a-month office visits until the most effective combination of drugs is found.

I cannot promise that our program will be 100 percent successful, as this is a very sick man, disabled for some years. However, there are some very positive indications—his determination to work on it, and his compliance with treatment.

Please give serious consideration to backing our program.

Sincerely yours,

Doctor's Name

SECOND REQUEST:

Some months later it became necessary to communicate again with the insurance company, to make sure the program could continue, with some modifications. The following letter tells the story.

DATE

TO: The patient's insurance company

Re: John Doe (the patient)

Address and social security number

Dear Administrator:

In the two months since my last report, I will have to add that Mr. Doe has been very faithful and compliant to the program I outlined in my letter of (date).

However, the program requires more visits for medication management and counseling by the psychiatrist than I had requested. I would change the request from once a month to weekly for a short time (one month), then to twice a month for one year.

Also, could the work of the therapist, the Rev. Richard Roe, LPC, be made retroactive to his contact?

Thanks for your consideration.

Sincerely Yours,

Doctor's Name

Appendix III
Annotated Bibliography

CHAPTER 1

American Psychiatric Association. (2001). The Treatment of Depressive Disorders—APA Symposium Highlights. *Psychiatric Annals*, Supplement. September. Washington, DC.

This supplement contains several important summaries described by Fawcett (p. 1) as follows:

> *In addition to an overview of depression and its pharmacology, the articles in this supplement provide information of various antidepressant types, a summary of some of the latest clinical studies regarding depressive disorders, and a review of treatment options. It also features articles specifically targeting the treatment of geriatric depression.*

Articles in the supplement that were not cited individually in the book itself but which may be of particular interest to readers of this book include the following:

Schatzberg, A. E. *New antidepressants may aid treatment of geriatric patients*. P. 1.

Alexopoulos, G. S. *Late-onset depression a predictor of poor treatment response in geriatric patients*. P. 2.

> *Poor treatment response appears to be a result of "depression executive dysfunction" syndrome, which occurs when the function of frontostriatal pathways is compromised.*

Katon, Wayne. *Collaborative care may improve patient remission rates*. P. 3.

A very good and detailed description of the problems of medically ill patients with depression and how much better the problems can be solved by cooperation and collaboration with the primary care physician.

> *Depression that is present with chronic medical illness causes added symptom burden, functional impairment, and decreased quality of life for these patients.*

Nelson, J. C. *Depression in the elderly may require more vigorous treatment over an extended duration*. P. 3.

Nelson gives specific details about medication, management, and types of response in the elderly that differ from other adults. He emphasizes the need to treat vigorously, probably with smaller doses of medication, to watch for side effects, and to expect that a longer time will be required for these cases. The psychosocial problems of the elderly, which contribute to the depression, are also emphasized.

Pollock, B. G. *Adverse drug reactions cause problems with depressive disorders.* P. 6.

A very thorough discussion of the physiological mechanism in these patients. Worth reading carefully.

> *. . . in terms of pharmacodynamic considerations, geriatric patients have a greater sensitivity to drugs, even at lower concentrations.*

Rapaport, M. H. *The societal impact of treating patients with depressive disorders.* P. 11.

The emphasis here is on "the dramatic change in the understanding of depression in terms of diagnosis, impact on a patient's quality of life, and long-term prognosis." He stresses the needs to treat the disability remaining after the symptoms are reduced, and not just the symptoms alone.

Kleiner, G. J., and Greston, W. M., eds. (1984). *Suicide in Pregnancy.* Bristol, London: John Wright PSG Inc.

CHAPTER 2

Akiskal, H. S., and Cassano, G. B., eds. (1997). *Dysthymia and the Spectrum of Chronic Depressions.* New York: Guilford Press.

A variety of contributors discuss primary dysthymia, chronic and residual major depressions, residual states in affective disorders and schizophrenic disorders, depressive personality, the concept of neurotic depression, neurasthenia and chronic fatigue, atypical depressions, brief depression, minor and recurrent, suicide, depression and attention-deficit/hyperactivity disorder, and chronic depression in childhood.

Angst, Jules. (1992). How recurrent and predictable is depressive illness? In *Long-Term Treatment of Depression. Perspectives in Psychiatry*, vol. 3. Edited by S. A. Montgomery and F. Rouillon. Chichester, England: John Wiley & Sons.

Single-episode depression is certainly less frequent than the estimate of 50 percent provided by several community studies would suggest. More recent prospective data indicate that only about *one quarter*, or even less, of all depressives are affected once in their lifetime. Today we can assume that 75 to 80 of cases are recurrent.

Recurrent depression mainly takes on the form of major depression and of recurrent brief depression. Major depression has a lifetime prevalence rate of 17 percent or more; recurrent brief depression of 11 percent or more. A prospective clinical study showed that recurrence of both unipolar depression and bipolar disorder does not diminish with age, but this finding needs further confirmation. Recurrence is difficult to predict. It is higher in bipolar disorders and in patients with early age of onset and with recurrent episodes prior to index episode. Future course is best predicted by the past course.

Contrary to recurrence, outcome (chronicity versus recovery) is influenced by numerous, probably additive factors, of which each may contribute a small amount to the variance. Comorbidity, multimorbidity, and the presence of physical disorders predict poor outcome, as does an inadequate, premorbid personality of maladjustment. To a probably minor extent other psychosocial factors may contribute; for instance, poor childhood care, lack of social support, the absence of a confidant, the presence of a sick partner, and strong expressed emotions in personal relationships.

Brugha, T. S. et al. (1997). Predicting the short-term outcome of first episodes and recurrences of clinical depression: A prospective study of life events, difficulties, and social support networks. *Journal of Clinical Psychiatry* 58(7):298–306.

High levels of adversity were related to a poor clinical course. Higher levels of social support predicted recovery from all but first episodes. There is progressive vulnerability to deficits in social supports with advancing course.

Coryell, William et al. (1994). The time course of nonchronic major depressive disorder. Uniformity across episodes and samples. *Archives of General Psychiatry* 51(5): 405–10.

Five participating centers conducted baseline assessments and followed 605 probands for up to 6 years. Forty percent recovered within 3 months; 60 percent recovered within 6 months; 80 percent recovered within one year; 20 percent had more protracted courses; 359 had at least one more episode; 181 had two episodes.

Gui, X-J., and Vaillant, G. E. (1997). Does depression generate negative life events? *Journal of Nervous and Mental Disease* 185:145–50.

A longitudinal study was done in 113 healthy Harvard graduates followed biennially from age 26 to age 62. Twelve men met criteria for affective disorder. This depressed group had a significantly higher density of dependent negative life events after the first episode of depression. The assumption is that having the depression generated self-induced negative life events, increasing the chronicity of the disorder and influencing the quality of life.

Lesse, Stanley, ed. (1974). *Masked Depression*. New York: Jason Aronson.

Montgomery, S. A., and Rouillon, F., eds. (1992).
Perspectives in Psychiatry, vol. 3: Long-Term Treatment of Depression. Chichester, England: John Wiley & Sons.

The authors believe that most of the depressive illnesses are recurrent, intermitted, or chronic. "We can assume that 75 to 80 percent of depressions are recurrent." There is a section on the complicated treatments required in both monopolar and bipolar illness. There is also a section on the usefulness of psychotherapy for prevention of relapse and recurrence.

Rush, A. J., and Thase, M. E. (1997). Strategies and tactics in the treatment of chronic depressions. *Journal of Clinical Psychiatry 58 (supplement 13)*: 14–22.

A good definition of chronicity: "Chronic depressions include major depressive disorder, recurrent, without full inter-episode recovery; major depressive disorder, currently in a chronic (i. e., > 2 years) episode; double depression; dysthymic disorder, and those depressive disorders—not otherwise specified (NOS)—that are persistent or predictably recurrent with substantial disability."

Solomon, D. A. et al. (1997). Recovery from major depression: a 10-year prospective follow-up across multiple episodes. *Archives of General Psychiatry* 54:1001–1006.

In this sample of patients treated at tertiary care centers for major depressive disorder, the duration of recurrent mood episodes was relatively uniform and averaged approximately 20 weeks. Sixty percent recovered within 6 months and 80 percent within one year from the later episodes, leaving 20 percent who took more than a year or became even more chronic.

Thase, M. E., and Howland, R. H. (1994). Refractory depression: relevance of psychosocial factors and therapies. *Psychiatric Annals* 24(5):232–40.

CHAPTER 4

Levitan, D. et al. (1998). Major depression in individuals with a history of childhood physical or sexual abuse: relationship to neurovegetative features, mania, and gender. *American Journal of Psychiatry* 155:12.

In the assessment of 8,116 individuals age 15 to 64, 653 cases of major depression were identified. A history of physical or sexual abuse in childhood was associated with major depression with reversed neurovegetative features, whether or not manic subjects were included in the analysis. A strong relationship between mania and childhood physical abuse was found. Across analyses there was a significant main effect of female gender on

risk of early sexual abuse; however, none of the
group-by-gender interactions predicted early abuse.

Tohen, Mauricio F. (1999). First-episode affective disorders with psychotic features: outcome. Syllabus
and Proceedings Summary of the Annual Meeting
of the American Psychiatric Association No. 29D,
p. 77. Washington, D.C.: American Psychiatric
Association.

Two-year outcome data for affective-disorder patients with psychosis. Two hundred and nineteen
patients were followed and evaluated for: (1) syndromal recovery and (2) functional recovery (vocational and residential status equal to or greater
than baseline). Syndromal recovery was reached
by 49 percent of patients within 3 months and 95
percent within 24 months. Functional recovery was
only 37 percent, and 63 percent of syndromally
recovered patients had not recovered functionally
within 2 years. (I include this summary because it
demonstrates that there is a large group of patients who need more for complete recovery than
the attention and treatment required to relieve the
immediate affective symptoms.

Weissman, M. M. (1997). Beyond symptoms: social
functioning and the new antidepressants. *Journal
of Psychopharmacology* 11 (Supplement): S5–S8.
———. (1999). Social functioning with the new treatments for depression. *Syllabus and Proceedings
Summary of the Annual Meeting of the American*

Psychiatric Association, p. 221. Washington, D.C.: American Psychiatric Association.

Depression scales assess the core biological features of the illness—mood, pessimism, and vegetative signs, (e.g., appetite and sleep loss). However, assessments of drive, motivation, performance, and quality of interpersonal relations (e.g., the social context once the symptoms are improved) may not be captured in the traditional symptom scales.

There is often a need for further treatment when the basic symptoms are controlled.

CHAPTER 5

Boyer, F. W., and Feighner, P. J. (1994). Clinical significance of early non-response in depressed. *Depression* 2:32–35.

In 6-week, double-blind control trials, if there is no improvement early in treatment, the chance of meaningful response by week 6 is poor. If the patient does not have at least 20 percent improvement in the HAMD score at any point during the first 4 weeks, the chance of the 6-week response is 3.7 percent.

Brown, C. et al. (1996). Treatment outcomes for primary care patients with major depression and lifetime anxiety disorders. *American Journal of Psychiatry* 153:1293–1300.

This randomized study compared the treatment response of depressed primary care patients with (107 patients) and without (50 patients) a lifetime anxiety disorder. Up to 60 percent of patients with major depression in psychiatric and primary care settings also suffer from comorbid anxiety or panic disorder. These patients have more severe depression, more suicidality and axis II diagnoses, and worse outcomes than patients with major depression alone. Fewer patients with comorbid depression and panic disorder had full recovery at 4 and 8 months, regardless of treatment modality.

Derogatis, R. L., and Wise, N. T. (1989). *Anxiety and Depressive Disorders in the Medical Patient*. Washington, D.C.: American Psychiatric Press.

Cassano, Giovanni, Savino, Mario, and Perugi, Giulio. (1992). Comorbidity of mood disorders and anxiety states. Implications for long-term treatment. In *Long-Term Treatment of Depression. Perspectives in Psychiatry*, vol. 3. Guilford, England: John Wiley & Sons.

There is substantial evidence of a less favorable outcome occurring among subjects with both anxiety and mood disorders, which would seem to underline the potential usefulness of the comorbidity concept.

Huxley, N. A., Parikh, S. V., and Baldessarini, R. J. (2000). Effectiveness of psychosocial treatments in bipolar disorder: state of the evidence. *Harvard Review of Psychiatry* 8(3):126–40.

P. 126: "Nevertheless, important gains were often seen, as determined by objective measures of increased clinical stability and reduced rehospitalization, as well as other functional and psychosocial benefits."

Johnson, F. N., ed. (1987). *Depression & Mania: Modern Lithium Therapy.* Oxford, England: IRL Press.

Excellent, even today, as we have not given up on lithium, despite newer drugs.

Kendler, K. S. et al. (1995). Stressful life events, genetic liability, and onset of an episode of major depression in women. *American Journal of Psychiatry* 152(6):833–42.

To illustrate, Kendler et al. (1995) studied more than a thousand female–female twin pairs to clarify how genetic liability and stressful events interact in the etiology of major depression. They found that while both genetic liability and stressful life events played roles in the onset of major depression during a given 30-day period, "the impact of stressful life events on the risk of onset of depression was much greater for individuals with high genetic liability [as suggested by a twin with a mood disorder] than for those at low genetic risk" in essence, genetic factors alter an individual's sensitivity to the "depressogenic" effects of stressful life events.

Mazur, Howard (1970). *People and Predicaments*. Cambridge, MA: Harvard University Press.

Meyersburg, H. A., and Post, R. M. (1979). An holistic developmental view of neural and psychological processes: a neurobiologic-psychoanalytic integration. *British Journal of Psychiatry* 135:139–55.

After a comprehensive review of the pertinent literature, the following conclusions are stated: "We postulate that environmental and social experiences may affect both the neural substrates and the subsequent behaviour which these neural structures subserve, given the particular state of development of the organism at the time. Environmental stress, such as severe deprivation or an overwhelming trauma, occurring during a vulnerable period, may evoke aberrant neuronal developmental patterns" (p. 150). "We postulate that there are biochemical, physiological, and neuroanatomical concomitants of what the psychoanalysts call fixation and regression. These may constitute the predisposition for the return to the earlier level of functioning" (p. 150). "We postulate that repetitive intense stresses or conflicts can be traumatic and have an impact in the infant similar to a subthreshold electrophysiological kindling process in the experimental animal" (p. 150). "We further postulate that these experiences of early psychological and (possibly) physiological "kindling" can result in the establishment of patterns of reaction in which distressing affect becomes magnified to the extent that the psychic functioning of the individual is disrupted, i.e., the psyche may become de-integrated and an episode of chaotic experience intervene. Such patterns may be re-invoked by a variety of adverse experiences in later life situations of the individual" (pp. 150–151).

Nemeroff, C. B. (1998). The neurobiology of depression. *Scientific American*, June, p. 48.

The persistence of the hyperactivity of neurosis in children activated by stress.

Nesse, R. M. (2000). Is depression an adaptation? *Archives of General Psychiatry* 57(1):14–20.

The author makes the point that the depression or low mood can be protective against something worse, yet it is also an illness with a great chance of suicide.

Olfson, M. et al. (1996). Subthreshold psychiatric symptoms in a primary care group practice. *Archives of General Psychiatry* 53(10):880–86.

Patients with a depressed mood or anhedonia for weeks, but without enough symptoms to qualify for a diagnosis of MDD, were 2.5 times more likely to have lost work or visited a mental health clinic, or to have had marital distress in the past month than patients without such symptoms, even after adjusting for the one third of patients in the subthreshold group with comorbid Axis I disorders (mostly drug abuse or dependence). Groups of patients with subthreshold depression and anxiety probably include some individuals with residual or prodromal MDD and PD and some with true partial syndromes. Although little formal research has been conducted on the treatment of subsyndromal conditions, the impairment they cause seems to justify intervention now and more research in the future.

Riddle, M. A. (1998). Efficacy of psychiatric medications in children and adolescents: a review of controlled studies. In *Psychiatric Clinics of North America: Annual of Drug Therapy*, pp. 269–85. Philadelphia: W. B. Saunders.

Up to 1998 only one drug, Prozac, had sufficient data to establish whether it was safe and/or effective for children with depression. *It was not found effective for treating depression in children.* It is essential to differentiate between prepubertal children and adolescents. Children in the adolescent years are highly susceptible to mood disorders whereas in pre-pubertal children one sees only the roots of the illnesses and the pre-illness symptoms.

Shneidman, S. E. (1976). *Suicidology: Contemporary Developments*. New York: Grune & Stratton.

The classic.

Strakowski, S. M. et al. (1998). Twelve-month outcome after a first hospitalization for affective psychosis. *Archives of General Psychiatry* 55(1):49–55.

Few patients achieved a favorable outcome in the year after a first hospitalization for an affective psychosis. Low socioeconomic status, poor premorbid function, treatment noncompliance, and substance abuse were associated with lower rates of delayed onset of recovery.

CHAPTER 6

American Psychiatric Association. (1994). Practice guidelines for the treatment of patients with bipolar disorder. *American Journal of Psychiatry* 151 (Supplement 12):1–36.

Two hundred fifty-six references.

Balon, Richard, and Riba, M. B. (2001). Improving the practice of split treatment. *Psychiatric Annals* 31 (10):582–628.

This is an entire issue devoted to issues relating to split treatment. The individual papers are:

Fawcett, Jan. Editorial: an issue that must be addressed. P. 582.

Balon, Richard. Positive and negative aspects of split treatment. Pp. 598–603.

Macbeth, J. E. Legal aspects of split treatment: how to audit and manage risk. Pp. 605–10.

Lazarus, J. A. Ethics in split treatment. Pp. 611–14.

Silk, K. R. Split (collaborative) treatment for patients with personality disorders. Pp. 615–22.

Himle, J. A. Medication consultation: the nonphysician clinician's perspective. Pp. 623–28.

Berman, R. M., Narasimhan, M., and Charney, D. S. (1997). Treatment-refractory depression: definitions and characteristics. *Depression and Anxiety* 5(4):154–64.

Entire issue devoted to the subject.

Blacker, D. (1996). Maintenance treatment of major depression: a review of the literature. *Harvard Review of Psychiatry* 4:1–9.

The literature shows that antidepressant medications and, to a lesser extent, psychotherapy are both effective in preventing recurrence of major depression. Maintenance treatment should be considered for a patient with recurrent major depression.

Calabrese, J. R. et al. (1993). Mixed states and bipolar rapid cycling and their treatment with Divalproex Sodium. *Psychiatric Annals* 23(2): 70–78.

An effective way to treat the 20 to 35 percent of patients who do not respond adequately to lithium.

Duckworth, Kenneth. (1998). Awakenings with the new antipsychotics. *Psychiatric Times Monograph*, December, pp. 26–27.

Points out the potential in patients on the new antipsychotic drugs for growth and maturation and for the elimination of long-standing malfunctions by psychotherapy once the symptoms of the illness (schizophrenia) are lessened or eliminated. This is a growing field because the new potent medications are getting more and more of the severely ill people well enough to focus on catching up with their emotional development. This factor is very evident in the mood disorders.

Evans, D. L. (1999). Assessing antidepressant efficacy: a reexamination. *Journal of Clinical Psychiatry* 60 (Supplement 4):3.

A substantial number of patients with depressive disorders do not respond completely to antidepressant treatment. Richard C. Shelton, M.D., reviews the options for dealing with nonresponsive, treatment-refractory patients. Although the time to response is often significantly delayed, most of these patients eventually remit.

Fenton, W. S., and McGlashan, T. H. (1997). We can talk: individual psychotherapy for schizophrenia. American Journal of Psychiatry 154:1493–95.

Fenton, W. S. (1998). Medication-psychotherapy combination most effective for schizophrenia. *Psychiatric Times Monograph* December, pp. 28–30.

Describes a disorder-specific individual psychotherapy called Personal Therapy characterized by flexibility first rigorously tested by a group in Pittsburgh. He quotes 2 papers:

Hogarty, G. E. et al. (1997). Three-year trials of personal therapy among schizophrenic patients living with or independent of family: I. Description of study and effects on relapse rates. *American Journal of Psychiatry* 154(11): 1504–13.

Hogarty, G. E. et al. (1997). Three-year trials of personal therapy among schizophrenic patients living with or independent of family: II. Effects on adjustment of patients. *American Journal of Psychiatry* 154(11): 1514–24.

Gabbard, G. O. (1992). Psychodynamic psychiatry in the "decade of the brain." *American Journal of Psychiatry* 149(8):991–98.

"Research on both primates and humans suggests that psychological influences result in permanent alterations of a neurobiological nature. Similarly, psychological interventions in a treatment context may have a profound impact on neurophysiology." Clinical understanding of the meaning of symptoms may be instrumental in ensuring patients' compliance with pharmacotherapy regimens and in the removal of other resistances to treatment. Conclusions: in contemporary psychiatry, a psychodynamic perspective must be preserved.

Hazell, D. P. et al. (1995). Efficacy of tricyclic drugs in treating child and adolescent depression: a meta-analysis. *British Medical Journal* 310:897–901.

A pooled analysis of 12 studies (146 patients and 157 controls) indicated that there was no significant benefit from active treatment (with drugs).

Judd, L. L. (1999). Treatment-resistant depression: guidelines for early diagnosis and recognition. *Syllabus and Proceedings Summary of the Annual Meeting of the American Psychiatric Association*, p. 223. Washington, DC: American Psychiatric Association.

There are three major goals in the treatment of major depressive episodes: (1) removal of depressive symptoms; (2) reduction or elimination of the associated impairment; and (3) the prevention of episode relapse or recurrence. Failure to achieve any or all of these treatment goals should be used to define treatment-resistant depression (TRD).

Keller, M. B. et al. (1998). Maintenance phase efficacy of sertraline for chronic depression: a randomized controlled trial. *Journal of the American Medical Association* 280(19):1665–72.

This was a study of 2 groups of patients: 1. Those with a diagnosis of chronic major depression (of at least 2 years' duration). 2. Patients with a diagnosis of dysthymia with a concurrent diagnosis of major depression (double depression). The diagnosis of "double depression" should be noted as it is a fairly common phenomenon, i.e., a person with dysthymia (formerly called neurotic depression) who develops a major depressive episode.

Kramer, P. D. (1993). *Listening to Prozac: A Psychiatrist Explores Antidepressant Drugs and the Remaking of the Self*. New York: Viking.

This introduced Prozac to the public, causing a remarkable expansion of its use. Very good bibliography. Also, the book introduced the idea that treatment by drugs can correct personality problems. Its great popularity seems largely due to the emphasis on how the drug can make people happier by appearing to treat personality deficiencies and disorders. Certain other antidepressant drugs can do the same, but this one is emphasized in this book. This effect on personality is a very controversial subject.

Kupfer, D. J. (1995). Acute continuation and maintenance treatment of mood disorders. *Depression* 3:137–38.

The phases of treatment are: acute, continuation, and maintenance. Most individuals will suffer recurrences, suggesting a need to develop long-term strategies. The continuation phase should last approximately 20 weeks if symptoms have remained in remission or recovery status has been reached. New studies show that medication should be continued at the same dose as in acute phase, and also throughout the maintenance phase (what gets you well keeps you well). Recently specific forms of psychotherapy have shown considerable efficacy not only for short-term treatments but also over the long term. We need to focus increasing attention on the adaptation of short-term treatment for the long term. Research is needed on combination treatments in both unipolar and bipolar disorders.

Maixner, S. M., and Greden, J. F (1998). Extended antidepressant maintenance and discontinuation syndromes. *Depression and Anxiety* 8 (Supplement 1):43–53.

Two different kinds of symptom clusters result from early discontinuation of the antidepressant medication. There can be either recurrence or relapse of the depression itself or "discontinuation syndrome" can occur, such as physical sensations of lightheadedness, dizziness, and vertigo. Noncompliance can be a cause of discontinuation, and it occurs sometimes because of the uncomfortable side effects, failure of supervision of the patient, failure to educate the patient in the use of medication, and necessity of long-term treatment.

Numerous studies demonstrate that maintenance antidepressants or mood-stabilizing medications are effective in preventing recurrences. All antidepressants are effective if full antidepressant doses are employed. If the patient discontinues abruptly, there will be unpleasant symptoms including dizziness, lightheadedness, electric-shock-like sensations, and gait instability. A gradual taper, perhaps extending for 3 to 6 months, can prevent this.

Montgomery, S. A., and Montgomery, D. B. (1992). Prophylactic treatment in recurrent unipolar depression. In *Long-Term Treatment of Depression. Perspectives in Psychiatry*, vol. 3. Guilford, England: John Wiley & Sons.

The results from these well-conducted studies provide a good scientific basis from the widely held clinical view that antidepressants, used in the long term, reduce the chances of new episodes of depression. Since depression is a highly recurrent disorder, the increased use of antidepressants in prophylaxis should reduce the overall morbidity.

Olfson, M., and Pincus, H. A. (1994). Outpatient psychotherapy in the United States, I. Volume, costs, and user characteristics. *American Journal of Psychiatry* 151:1281–88.

Rogers, W. H. et al. (1993). Outcomes for adult outpatients with depression under prepaid or fee-for-service financing. *Archives of General Psychiatry* 50(7): 317–25.

Samuels, S. C., and Katz, I. B. (1995). Depression in the nursing home. *Psychiatric Annals* 25(7):419–24.

Schore, N. A. (1994). *Affects Regulation and the Origin of the Self: Neurology of Emotional Development*. Hillsdale, NJ: Lawrence Erlbaum Associates.

Shelton, R. C. (1999). Treatment options for refractory depression. *Journal of Clinical Psychiatry* 60 (Supplement 4):57–61.

A significant proportion of patients with depressive disorders does not experience a full response with antidepressant treatment. Fortunately, most eventually remit, even though the time to response may be significantly delayed in many patients. A variety of options exist to deal with these difficult clinical situations. Established strategies include switching to an antidepressant of an alternative class (e.g., tricyclic to a monoamine oxidase inhibitor [MAOI] or selective serotonin reuptake inhibitor [SSRI], electroconvulsive therapy (ECT), and augmentation with lithium or thyroid hormone. Promising alternatives include combined serotonin and norepiphrine enhancement strategies (e.g., SSRI plus serotonin norepinephrine reuptake inhibitor [NSRI] or higher doses of venlafaxine or fluoxetine), steroid suppression therapy, augmentation therapy, augmentation with atypical antipsychotics, and psychotherapy.

Sherwood B. E., and Suppes, T. (1998). Bipolar disorders. *Psychiatric Clinics of North America: Annual of Drug Therapy*, pp. 145–60. Philadelphia: W. B. Saunders.

A review of a lifelong management of both mania and depression with a list of 140 references up to and including 1997.

Soumerai, S. B. et al. (1994). Effects of limiting Medicaid drug-reimbursement benefits on the use of psychotropic agents and acute mental health services by patients with schizophrenia. *New England Journal of Medicine* 331(10):650–55.

Limiting Medicaid drug costs resulted in a drop in cost of $5.14 per patient per month for drugs, but visits to community mental health centers rose by about $139 per patient per month. It was estimated that the cost of services was about 17 times greater than the savings.

Stahl, S. M. (1998). Basic psychopharmacology of antidepressants, part I. Antidepressants have several distinct mechanisms of action. *Journal of Chemical Psychiatry* 59 (Supplement 4):5–14.

The antidepressants can be separated into several distinct classes on the basis of distinct pharmacological mechanisms. These are:

Tricyclic antidepressants: imipramine, norpramine, amitriptyline, nortriptyline

Monoamine Oxidase Inhibitors (MAO inhibitors): parnate, nardil

Selective Serotonin Reuptake Inhibitors (SSRIs): (Prozac) fluoxetine, sertraline (Zoloft, paroxetine (Paxil)

Selective Serotonin Reuptake Inhibitors with other actions.

Also

a. norepinephrine reuptake inhibitors: (neurofaxin) (Effexor)

b. Serotonin-2 antagonism reuptake inhibitors: (nefazadone) (Serzone)

c. Alpha antagonism plausiseratonin-2 and 3-antagonism: (mirtazepine) (Remeron)

Selective norepinephrine and dopamine reuptake inhibitor bupropion with no action on the serotonin systems: (Wellbutrin).

Thase, M. E., and Rush, A. J. (1995). Treatment-resistant depression. In *Psychopharmacology: The Fourth Generation of Progress*. New York: Raven Press.

SSRI drugs seem to produce lower average sleep efficiency, whereas trazodone (Desyrel) and nefazadone (Serzone) augment sleep.

———. (1997). When at first you don't succeed: sequential strategies for antidepressant nonresponders. *Journal of Clinical Psychiatry* 58 (Supplement 13): 23–29.

For depressed patients who did not benefit with first line of antidepressant agents, alternate antidepressant strategies as a 5-stage strategy progressing from simpler such as alternate monotherapy to more complex strategies, combination or augmentation regimens, with nonselective monoamine oxidase inhibitors (+/– lithium salts) and electroconvulsive therapy reserved for treatment stages III and IV. Psychotherapeutic management also is an important ingredient in the ongoing treatment of these patients, particularly to counteract the demoralization and frustration accompanying the failure to respond.

CHAPTER 7

Abraham. Karl. (1948). *Selected Papers on Psycho-Analysis*. London: Hogarth Press and The Institute of Psycho-Analysis.

Akiskal, H. S. (1992). Psychopharmacological and psychotherapeutic strategies in intermittent and chronic affective conditions. In *Long-Term Treatment of Depression. Perspectives in Psychiatry*, vol. 3. Guilford, England: John Wiley & Sons.

The long-term psychopharmacological management of this very complex group of chronic patients is still very much of an art that each clinician must develop by informed "trial and error" on a large number of patients examined over long periods of personal follow-up. Such experience will teach the physician that psycho-educational and psychotherapeutic approaches can considerably enhance the gains made through chemotherapy.

Clemens, N. A. (2000). Review of "Psychotherapy indications and outcomes edited by David S. Janowsky, Washington, D.C. American Psychiatric Press." *Psychiatric Services* 52:683.

Clemens does more than just review the book on psychotherapy medications and outcomes. He also gives the reader useful insights into the present state of acceptance of the various methods pf psychotherapy used today—a valuable summary indeed.

Dietrich, R. D., and Shabad, C. P. (1989). *The Problem of Loss and Mourning: Psychoanalytic Perspectives*. Madison, WI: International University Press.

Frank, Ellen, Johnson, Sheri, and D. J. Kupfer. (1992). Psychological treatment in prevention of relapse. In *Long-Term Treatment of Depression. Perspectives in Psychiatry*, vol. 3. Guilford, England: John Wiley & Sons.

Overall, then, the field of psychotherapy research in depressive disorders has witnessed enormous advances in methodological sophistication and increasing attention (p. 224) to long-term outcome. Results of these efforts have been promising across several different forms of psychotherapy. Despite significant advances, conclusions have been limited by the small number of studies and a series of methodological problems. The most pervasive methodological difficulties have included a failure *to report treatment specificity*, inadequate provision of medication, most frequently in the form of abrupt withdrawal, analyses of discrete points in time rather than cumulative probability of relapse, and small sample sizes. Despite these problems, one conclusion emerges across a range of studies. As is the case with pharmacotherapy, continuing psychotherapy after initial recovery is a powerful technique in the prevention of relapse and recurrence.

Gaylin, Willard, ed. (1968). *The Meaning of Despair*. New York: Jason Aronson.

Gottschalk, A. L. (1989). *How to Do Self-Analysis and Other Self-Psychotherapies*. Northvale, NJ: Jason Aronson.

Excellent description of the self-analysis that typically can be done after a personal analysis. Also, describes a method of self-analysis originated by the author.

Greenacre, Phyllis, ed. (1953). *Affective Disorders: Psychoanalytic Contribution to Their Study*. New York: International Universities Press.

Jacobson, Edith. (1971). *Depression: Comparative Studies of Normal, Neurotic, and Psychotic Conditions*. New York: International Universities Press.

An insightful study of what lies behind the symptoms, and who responds to psychodynamic therapy.

Lewin, D. B. (1950). *The Psychoanalysis of Elation*. New York: W. W. Norton.

A classic description of the psychology of elation in the manic disorder as seen in psychoanalytic studies.

Lindemann, Erich. (1979). *Beyond Grief: Studies in Crisis Intervention*. New York: Jason Aronson.

Again, a classic early description of the course and therapy of mourning, but the first to present insights into grief and mourning as a process.

Loewenstein, M. R., ed. (1953). *Drives, Affects, Behavior*. New York: International University Press.

Psychoanalytic papers on the work of several experts in the field of depression. Very important in representing the insights of what lies behind the symptoms.

Meredith, L. S. (1996). Counseling typically provided for depression. Role of clinician specially specialty and payment system. *Archives of General Psychiatry* 53:905–12.

A survey by *Consumer Reports* found that people who received psychotherapy from mental health professionals were more satisfied than people who received psychotherapy from primary care physicians.

Mitscherlich, Alexander, and Mitscherlich, Margarete. (1975). *The Inability to Mourn: Principles of Collective Behavior*. New York: Grove Press.

Scott, W. I. D. (1962). Hamlet, the manic depressive. In *Shakespeare's Melancholics*, pp. 73–107. London: Mills and Boon.

I don't agree that Hamlet was a manic depressive. He was a victim of grief from an act that needed revenge. A grief that was complicated and atypical.

Excellent description of the psychology of the German people after World War II.

Seligman, E. P. M. (1975). *Helplessness: On Depression, Development, and Death*. San Francisco: W. H. Freeman.

A classic description of helplessness, an affect that lies behind many depressions as first described by Edward Bibring in his article, "The mechanism of depression," in *Affective Disorders*, ed. P. Greenacre, pp. 13–48. New York: International Universities Press.

Winson, J. (1990). The meaning of dreams. *Scientific American*, November, pp. 48–57.

From neurophysiological research, Winson concludes, "For reasons that he could not possibly have known, Freud set forth a profound truth in his work. There is an unconscious, and dreams are indeed the 'royal road' to its understanding. However, the characteristics of the unconscious and associated processes of brain functioning are very different than Freud thought. Rather than being a cauldron of untamed passion and destructive wishes, I propose that the unconscious is a cohesive, continually active mental structure that takes note of life's experiences and reacts accordingly to its own scheme of interpretation."

Wylie, H. W., Jr., and Wylie, M. L. (1987). An effect of pharmacotherapy on the psychoanalytic process:

case report of a modified analysis. *American Journal of Psychiatry* 144(4):489-92.

CHAPTER 8

Beers, W. C. (1981). *Mind that Found Itself*. Pittsburgh: University of Pittsburgh Press.

The first description by the patient of his own bipolar illness, and how he felt throughout the course of it.

Cammer, Leonard. (1969). *Up from Depression*. New York: Pocket Books.

Hampton, K. R. (1975). *The Far Side of Despair: A Personal Account of Depression*. Chicago: Nelson-Hall.

Hellmuth, F. C. (1977). *Manic: Anatomy of Mental Illness*. Philadelphia: Dorrance & Company.

Jamison, K. R. (1995). *An Unquiet Mind: A Memoir of Moods and Madness*. New York: Vintage Books.

A remarkably candid look by a gifted woman who describes her experience of having bipolar illness and yet managed to have a successful career after a period of several cycles before conquering the disease. She also co-authored the classic modern book on manic-depressive illness. The *New England Journal of Medicine* called it a "must read." The *British Medical Journal* called it a "landmark."

Kraines, H. S., and Thetford. S. E. (1972). *Help for the Depressed*. Springfield, IL: Charles C. Thomas.

LaHaye, T. (1974). *How to Win Over Depression*. Grand Rapids, MI: Zondervan.

Logan, Joshua. (1976). *Josh: My Up and Down, In and Out Life*. New York: Delacorte Press.

The autobiography of probably one of the most successful theater directors of all times on the New York Stage. He suffered from bipolar disorder, and gives an intimate description from the inside of what it is like to go through the experience of being manic, and then of being depressed and getting electroshock therapy. Most interesting is the obvious fact that he was unaware that he was ill or had changed in his behavior, and someone had to step in and rescue him.

It is also very helpful in giving a description of the problem personality that is sometimes behind the illness, especially in gifted, bright, and successful persons. There is also a description of the kind of traumatic childhood of the illness, plus the revelation, near the end of the book, that his father had committed suicide.

This book clearly shows how undiagnosed illness complicated his life, but also how creative and productive a gifted hypomanic person can be. It is an example of how the illness does not always prevent a person from being very successful in our society, if properly handled. Worth reading for patients, families, and professionals.

Medina, John. (1998). *Depression: How it Happens, How it's Healed.* Oakland, California: New Harbinger Publications and CME.

A popular book by a psychologist (not a psychiatrist!) who is a molecular biologist and a professional writer for the *Psychiatric Times*. Its 146 pages are beautifully illustrated, and understandable to both laypersons and general medical practitioners. The author is not biased toward any one treatment method but gives an objective view of pharmacological, psychosocial, and psychotherapeutic interventions. The diagrams, tables, and illustrations alone are very helpful. There are some shortcomings. For example, children receive too little space, the summary on children is too vague, and although it does distinguish childhood depression from the adult form it specifically leaves out any definitive approach to treatment. Also it fails to distinguish adolescence from childhood.

Peabody, W. F. (1930). *Doctor and Patient.* New York: Macmillan.

A classic description of the physician-patient relationship.

Rosen, L. E., and Amador, X. F. (1996). *When Someone You Love is Depressed: How to Help Your Loved One Without Losing Yourself.* New York: The Free Press.

This book goes into some details about recognizing the illness in a family member, and about how to live with such a member when treatment is going on. There are details, such as the way to deal with different family members—parent, partner, a child. There is a description of communicating with depressed persons, and treatments are also included—drugs psychological treatments, and their dangers, including suicide.

Weissman, M. M., and Paykel, E. S. (1974). *A Depressed Woman: A Study of Social Relationships*. Chicago: University of Chicago Press.

Index

children, pharmacotherapy
for, 239, 243–244
chronic depression. *See*
chronicity
chronicity, 5–9, 11–13, 24–29,
44–47, 104–105. *See also*
depression; Multiaxial
System
causes of, 62–64
clinical description of
patients, 20–21
defined, 15–20, 207–208, 231
frequency of, 31–33, 186, 187
identifying causes of, 47–48
negative factors contributing
to, 58–59
positive factors contributing
to, 61, 66–67
quality of life (QOL) problems and, 46
recovery *vs.*, 229
spectrum disorders and, 46
subsynchromal symptomatic
depression, 46
Ciechanowski, P.S., 108–109
Clemens, N.A., 251–252
clinical disorders, personality
disorders *vs.*, 68–71
clomipramine hydrochloride,
147, 214
clonazepam, 173
clozapine, 164, 173
Clozaril. *See* clozapine
cognition, 70
Cognitive-Behavioral Analysis
System (CBAS), 120, 122–
126, 129, 205

cognitive therapy, 98, 116–117,
119–120
Commission on Professional
and Hospital Activities
2001, 24
comorbidity, 23, 48, 50–52,
203, 234–235
Consumer Reports, 254
continuation phase, of treatment, 131–134, 136–137
Coryell, William, 230

dehydroindolone, 218
Delgado, Pedro L., 114–15,
199–200
Depakote. *See* divalproex
sodium
dependency, 107–108
depression. *See also* chronicity;
pharmacotherapy;
*individual names of
depressive disorders*
atypical, 162
depressive personality
disorder, 22
early non-response in, 234
genetic liability and, 236
interpersonal *vs.* intrapersonal aspects of,
128–129
latent, 25–29
major depressive disorder
(MDD), 16, 44–45,
187–188, 230
negative life events and, 230
recurrent, 228–229
supervision for, 37
Depression, 204, 234, 245–246

negative factors, 61, 66–67
applied retroactively, 170
case studies using, 157–158
Nelson, J.C., 226–227
Nemeroff, C.B., 206
Nesse, R.M., 48
neurobiology
holistic developmental view
of, 237–238
monoamine depletion and
depression, 199–200
neurochemistry and, 95–97
permanent alterations to, 243
neuroses, 23–24
*New England Journal of
Medicine*, 248–249
New Yorker, 115
non benzodiazepine hypnotics,
216
norepinephrine, 114, 200, 249

Oates, Joyce Carol, 57–60
obsessive-compulsive disorder
(OCD), 147
Olfson, M., 238–239
O'Reardon, J.P., 20

Parikh, S.V., 235–236
passivity, 11
patients. *See also* medical
doctors; Multiaxial
System; therapists
chronic, 20–21 (*See also*
chronicity)
hospitalized, 207
long-term, 8
10-year follow-up study of,
38–42

25-year follow-up study of,
33–38, 41–42
personality disorders
clinical disorders *vs.*, 68–71
defined, 70–71
depressive, 22
intimate relationships
and, 6–9 (*See also*
predicament)
origin of personality
attributes, 146
predicament and, 121–122
reoccurrence and, 54–55
Personal Therapy, 130, 179
Perspectives in Psychiatry,
228–229, 231, 235, 247,
252–253
Perugi, Giulio, 235
pharmacotherapy, 68–69, 114–
115, 138–142, 147, 213.
See also chronicity; comorbidity; doctor-patient
relationship; neurobiol-
ogy; treatment; *individual
drug classes; individual
drug names*
adverse reactions to, 227
Anna Freud on, 127
antidepressant study, 247
antipsychotic drugs, 242
appropriateness of, 195
for atypical depression, 162
for children, 239, 243–244
Clemens on, 252
combined methods of
psychotherapy and,
94–95, 116–117

About the Author

Daniel W. Badal, M.D. began his research in clinical and laboratory work on depression and other mood disorders at the Massachusetts General Hospital and the Harvard Medical School, and later at the Medical School of the Case Western Reserve University and at the School of Social Work. He continues teaching residents and medical students at Case Western Reserve Medical School. In 1999, Dr. Badal was awarded the American Psychiatric Association Tenth Annual Nancy C.A. Roeske, M.D. Certificate of Recognition for Excellence in Medical Student Teaching. He also teaches on the psychology and psychodynamics of mood disorders and on the use of medication in combination with psychotherapy and psychoanalysis to analytic candidates at the Cleveland Psychoanalytic Institute.